MW01204219

7 Steps to Healing and Wellness

7 Steps
to Healing and
Wellness

Using Essential Oils
And the Kybalion as a guide

BY

Nalani D. Valentine, CND, PhD

HEAL BY TOUCH PUBLICATIONS, NEW YORK

ISBN: 978-0-6151-7618-5

In 1996, Dr. Nalani was diagnosed with breast cancer. She healed herself, using the same principles that are in this book, without the use of pharmaceutical medication, or drugs of any type, and has been cancer-free ever since.

The above statement is not intended for any purpose other than to relate a personal experience.

This book is dedicated:

To my father, Sampson Thaddeus Horton; though you made your transition years ago, you are forever with me.

To my mother, Mildred Arthelia White; always a lady, you taught me unconditional love. You told me I could do anything; and I believed you.

To all my ancestors including Nathaniel Turner; thank you for your indomitable blood in my veins, and for your constant encouragement.

Acknowledgments

My gifted and beautiful daughters—inside and out—Camille, Nanette, Mazz and Allisyn; and to my grandchildren, nieces and nephews; I love you deeply.

Camille Horton - my only sister, thank you for always being there for me, and for designing my book covers.

Ronald Swift - my former husband of 32 good years, thank you for selflessly providing through all those years.

My brothers - Sampson, David—thank you for your help—Nicholas and Stephen; I love you all.

Dr. Phillip Valentine, Senu Aakhu Ra Imhotep El, Mry, My polarity, the gentle nurturer nobody knows like I do; thank you for your love, encouragement and editing.

Junior Coggins - thank you for your illustrations and your patient assistance.

Dr. Gary and Mary Young - Thank you for your dedication to the integrity of Young Living Essential Oils.

Portions of this book are extrapolated from my more in-depth work entitled The Metaphysics of Health and Healing.

 As you explore the following principles, you will find a few simple exercises to help you internalize the essence of each one. You will also learn of specific Essential Oils that will help you to resonate on the same frequencies as the principles listed.

Addendum

Since this book was first written 2 years ago, there has been a serious setback in the Health Care Community. For more than 10 years now, we have been warned that the FDA (the government Food and Drug Administration) backed by the Codex Alimentarius Commission (established in 1963 by 2 international interests: the World Health Organization (WHO), and the Food and Agriculture Organization (FAO) was moving toward abrogating our lawful right to use vitamins, herbs and other natural supplements here in the United States.

While as a Hygienic Naturopath, I don't necessarily recommend the use of herbs and vitamins, unless in extreme cases, and in the case of an emergency, I absolutely support our right to use them.

According to the Codex Commission's web site, the "main purposes of this Programme are protecting the health of the consumers and ensuring fair trade practices in the food trade, and promoting coordination of all food standards work undertaken by international governmental and non-governmental organizations."

These are obviously very viable and necessary aspirations. Yet as we all well know, the Commission allows extremely dangerous and toxic drugs to be approved for public consumption—even when serious complications and even death can KNOWINGLY be the result.[i]

Although the subject of protecting and preserving our remaining rights is of paramount import, it is

---

[i] See the Internet documentary on Codex "We become Silent" by Kevin Miller

not what this book is about. This book was written to aid the reader in realizing and maintaining optimum health—not to be a political catalyst. But now, as I re-write in July of 2006, the FDA has added Essential Oils to the category listing of "drugs". This move has far-reaching global implications that now make it necessary for me to insert a stronger, more detailed disclaimer regarding therapeutic grade Essential Oils, even though I know their value from years of research, and experience with clients, as well as personal use.

Disclaimer

The FDA does not recognize the practice of Aromatherapy or the use of Essential Oils; neither has it evaluated any statements regarding Essential Oils herein.

No information in this book (including the technical scientific facts) is intended as medical advice, or to diagnose or treat any illness, condition or disease.

If you are pregnant, nursing or have a chronic illness, seek professional advice before using Essential Oils. Dilute one part Essential Oil with one part vegetable oil. If irritation occurs, do not use water; use vegetable oil to cleanse the area, and wipe dry.

Keep Essential Oils away from young children and away from the eyes.

CONTENTS

INTRODUCTION

"When the ears of the student are ready to hear, then come the lips to fill them with wisdom"
- The Kybalion

The Kybalion was compiled and written by The Three Initiates. It is a book of the 7 Hermetic Principles of Life. These principles were named after the Master of masters, teacher Hermes Trismegistus or, 'The Thrice Great' - whose origin as Djehuti can be traced back to the African land of Kemet (later re-named Aegyptos, or Egypt by the Greeks).

The Hermetic Principles were originally not written; rather, they were passed verbally from master to initiate, because as the Initiates put it, the Masters "knew the folly of attempting to teach the world that which it was neither ready nor willing to receive".

The Kybalion is a simply written and easily read book of aphorisms—fundamental truths, taught as far back as 10 millennia ago. It is not a religious work, but you will find many of those ancient and eternal truths in the doctrines and philosophies of every religion today.

For centuries, mastering the mental forces of the mind has been the goal and aspiration of many who not only hunger for knowledge and truth, but who also diligently and unceasingly search for the elusive answers to the mysteries of life. Careful study of the Kybalion is an important first step toward achieving that goal.

When understood, innerstood and adhered to, the 7 Kemetic/Hermetic principles of the Kybalion give insight and guidance to the seeker's search for truth, by lifting the veil of ambiguity from his or her consciousness.

I have integrated these 7 Principles into an approach to Healing and the realization of Wellness that I am pleased to share with you in the following pages.

The 7 Principles of the Kybalion

1. **Mentalism** - All is mind; the Universe is mental

2. **Correspondence** - As above so below, as below so above

3. **Vibration** - All that takes form vibrates

4. **Polarity** – Everything is dual; everything has its poles

5. **Rhythm** – Everything flows out and in; everything has its tides

6. **Cause and Effect** – For every action there is an equal and opposite reaction

7. **Gender** – Gender is in everything; everything has its masculine and feminine principles

Fear less, hope more; eat less, chew more; whine less, breathe more; talk less, say more; hate less, love more; and all good things are yours.

\- Swedish Proverb

The Seven Steps

1. Mindful Living
2. Agreement
3. Resonance
4. Equilibrium
5. Flow of Life
6. Karma
7. Posterity

"Be careful about reading health books. You may die of a misprint"

- Mark Twain

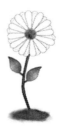

Chapter One

An Overview

THE WORD "WELLNESS" HAS BECOME a popular
term for good health. It's more than just the
absence of physical pain, or the exhibition of
strength. It infers the harmony between the
psycho-spiritual and emotional bodies as well.

When you are well, all is balanced in your world,
and nothing has the power to move you too far
from that state. Your consciousness rests in a
space of equilibrium; you feel good. You feel good
because all of your checks and balances have
been literally checked and balanced. Every
aspect of your being—from your astral body to
the dense callus on the bottom of your feet as the

living hologram of the complete you—is vibrating in synchronicity; harmonious existence with your inner and outer worlds causes you to feel lighter, without the sensation of cumbersome weights of any form.

When you are not feeling well you have been moved to a space of imbalance—for example when you are angry—you are cosmically participating in the illusion of fragmentation. In other words, you are no longer functioning in your world as a being that is one with the world. Instead, you feel a sense of separation; you are feeling alone. This is indeed an illusion because there is no way that you can be truly alone. It is a matter of perception (as everything is). Your envelope of consciousness, though distinctly aware of the "personal self", cannot be separated or polarized, but it is the powerful effect of a repetitious thought-loop based on isolation that re-enforces the illusion of separation, and makes it appear real. It's the affect of a romance-consciousness that is invoked and developed for example, by love songs, novels and movie themes.

The problem is that we in the western world have come to believe our own fantasies. We not only escape to the TV and to movies, but we allow the fictitious entities to escape the theaters and go home with us—to move into our indelible psyches, and begin to influence our thought patterns, and thus our daily lives.

Music composed for the movies is designed to invoke deep emotional feelings of empathy for the characters in the story being portrayed. It is designed to reach into the soul of the viewer, where it may leave a false imprint of loneliness that we passively accept. But in reality, with each breath we take, we are sharing with each other and with everything else the atomic substances that help to keep us alive and well.

You are not alone.

You can exist in a perpetual state of wellness.

Many who seek higher consciousness have reached a level where they don't allow anything or anyone to dictate the way they feel. It's not that they are apathetic, but they fully understand that this existence is an illusory pact of agreements, and everything that they participate in is based on *choice.*

Some have found the wellness state of mind while their physical bodies are approaching imminent death on a hospital bed. They are the ones who smile at you from the opposite end of your empathic tears; they know. They know inner peace; they know unconditional love. They know what reality is, as opposed to the illusion of this present mundane physical existence. They accept and surrender to the "now" and don't fret about "yesterday" or "tomorrow".

Wellness also implies the sublime expression of Divine[1] intent.

Before you were born, you projected and solidified your intent to live and to grow on the physical planes of existence. That intent vibrates on a level of consciousness that we may seldom pay

---

[1]Don't be intimidated by the word. Divine simply means "very good" or "the most good". To some, it means "of God".

attention to, but nevertheless is a major aspect of our being.

Nobody's perfect; right? Wrong!

"Our body is a machine for living. It is organized for that, it is its nature. Let life go on in it unhindered and let it defend itself, it will do more than if you paralyze it by encumbering it with remedies."

~Leo Tolstoy

Somewhere along the way you were made to believe that you were less than perfect. At first, it may have been parents or other family members who molded your perceptions to believe you were lacking. During your pre-school days, you watched cartoons and commercials on TV where a certain look was portrayed as beautiful, handsome or strong; a different look was depicted as ugly, weak and even laughable, and only a particular "type" with a specific "look" was considered socially acceptable to be looked upon with respect.

Then you went to school. Other children burdened with their own learned insecurities and self-doubts teased, laughed and confirmed and helped to solidify your less-than-perfect self-image, and through the years your insecurities grew as you grew.

Just as you learned to listen to outside voices, you can learn to recognize your own true inner voice. This is the voice that accepts and appreciates your SELF in every aspect. It reflects and expresses your original intent to exist. It doesn't know lack; it simply acknowledges all.

Initially as children we knew that inner voice well. It's just that we listened to all voices with the same degree of acceptance, and we gradually learned to respect outside voices above our own.

14

Movies, songs, Ken & Barbie dolls, school books, magazines and popular trends provided more images to compare yourself with, and you were convinced that you were "less than". After all, these images never seemed to have any flaws; they spoke loudly with the same voice, so "they" must have been right. Even the giant pictures on the sides of buildings and buses agreed; they all screamed... "You are NOT perfect!"

Beloved, know that you are a creation of the Most High Creator. The Most High, as the purest expression of absolute perfection, makes no mistakes. Maybe you were taught that only God is perfect.

But is there anywhere that God is not God?

When we realize and accept that we are perfect even with our imperfections, is when we begin to recognize the inner voice of truth; and then, with those childhood voices silent, we begin the outward expression of the wellness state.

The nutritional choices we make, the supplementations we choose, and the essential oils we may use are all secondary and tertiary elements that are added to the more crucial metaphysical templates we create.

Cognitive and internal nutritional interplay can be very subjective. The result of this exchange can express itself as a heavy ball-&-chain type burden, insistently lurking in the back of your mind, periodically re-surfacing to the forefront to remind you of what you "should" or "shouldn't" be eating.

Equally verifiable is the fact that while one person is constantly worrying about "eating right", yet gets "sick" often, another can eat "anything and everything in sight", and seemingly not experience any negative repercussions.

Overstanding the power and the workings of intent, thought, and subconscious agreements with the intelligence in and of individual physiology, we can realize that this phenomenon is really not such a paradox after all. We each express health in our own unique way. Strong, healthy metaphysical templates can often override or nullify the consequences of unhealthy eating—for a time, but eventually, the effects of such eating will become evident.

Nutritional supplements can be good—and even necessary at times, but we need to be aware of the underlying causal factors that make them necessary, and then work toward permanently eliminating them.

Throughout this book, you will hear me repeatedly say that Essential Oils are very helpful, but they won't heal you. My mantra has been, and will continue be, "you heal yourself".

As you read, take your time. Feel free to use this as a workbook; take advantage of the extra spaces and blank pages to jot down your own relevant thoughts.

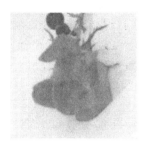

Chapter 2
Therapeutic Grade Essential Oils

There is NOTHING that you can ingest that will heal you. Essential Oils (EO's), vitamins, "super foods", "power juices", herbs, tonics and drugs notwithstanding, **you heal you, period.**

Contrary to popular belief, substances do not "act" on the body. Whenever a substance is ingested, your body must act upon *it!* If you were to take a drug, herb, EO or vitamin and somehow place it in a lifeless body, nothing would happen—except that the EO may help to preserve whatever portion of the tissues it came into contact with. Other than that, there would be no interaction between the substance and the body. But put a drug or any other substance in a living being and all sorts of activity immediately ensues!

It all depends on what the substance calls for. Some substances require the body to use more energy than others, as it determines what action to take, but again, it is the living body that acts on the drug—not the other way around.

Innate Divine Intelligence, as we will see later, is diligently and vigilantly working to maintain optimum health and vitality. It will do whatever is immediately necessary—sometimes expending much energy—to restore internal balance.

Ah, me! Love can not be cured by herbs.

- Ovid

Your body recognizes sunlight, oxygen, water and nutritious food as necessary components for sustenance. They require the least effort to metabolize. **Anything** else will trigger a defense response.

A symptom is not a disease! It is a signal that lets you know that something is out of balance. One should think about that when watching the overly abundant, skillfully orchestrated commercials that are constantly played on TV. Think of inner intelligence, warning you that something is not as it should be, and of the very possible *future consequence* of you telling that intelligence to "shut up, go away, don't warn me, don't tell me anything, I just want to feel good now."

Drugs and most herbs re-direct energy from pathological symptoms, by insidiously—and sometimes overtly creating a secondary pathological condition, quietly extracting vitality from essential body organs.

Herbs are closer in substance to foods, and therefore can be less threatening at times, but the body still does not recognize them as food.

Obviously there are times of emergency when drugs are absolutely necessary, but we should not be so quick to make them the first and only avenue to take when the body is giving warning symptoms.

Therapeutic grade Essential Oils are oxygen carriers, and do not require digestion. Not only do they oxygenate the blood, but they also assist the body in transferring oxygen through the cellular wall and into the cells where it is needed. For this and other reasons, practitioners who have studied EO's tend to be enthusiastic when recommending them. They know their potential; they have witnessed their power to assist the body in removing obstacles to healing. **Still, Essential Oils will not heal you.**

Essential oils are volatile substances that are extracted from different parts of a plant. Most citrus oils are pressed from the rind; according to the particular plant, some oils are distilled from the flowers, stem or root. These oils are very complex; they contain numerous chemical elements that interact with human and animal metabolism. It is the molecular structure of the oils that make them particularly effective as healing agents. They have a similar and compatible molecular structure to that of our blood cells, rendering them easily recognized and assimilated by the body (not as food, but as the chemical gases that our food is ultimately converted into).

Red blood cells (erythrocytes) carry oxygen and nutrients to every part of the human body. Essential oils carry plant-nutrients throughout the plant, and function as its chemical defense mechanism. They also transport oxygen and nutrients through the cellular membranes of our bodies, as they do of the plant.

Each plant species has its unique assortment of from 80 to more than 300 constituents that differentiates its oil from the others, and even within each category, there are biochemically unique variants (chemotypes). Essential Oils that are extracted from these plants can have several thousand constituents.

Therapeutic EO's do not shock or force the body to respond. As mentioned before, they bring oxygen and other supportive components of the blood into the cells. In this manner they are "used up" by the body, and do not accumulate therein.

Not all Essential Oils are created equal. There are several factors that come together to create Therapeutic Grade oils:

- The primary constituents of the oil have to be present in specific percentages
- the original plant must be organically grown

- the quality and quantity of nutrients in the soil that the plant was grown in must be high
- The distillery should be stainless steel—not aluminum or copper, which are reactive
- the crop must be harvested at the optimal time for the plant
- the oil must be distilled slowly, at a low temperature, and
- the oil should **not be mixed** or cut with any other chemicals.

An Essential Oil can be analyzed by a specially trained chemist who understands the intricacies of a gas chromatograph chart, where she can examine its entire chemical imprint, for purity and potency. Very few companies that process essential oils are willing to spend the additional time and resources required to meet these standards.

Adulterated and otherwise less-than-therapeutic grade Essential Oils can be harmful at the most, (causing burn, rashes, allergic reactions, etc.) and just plain ineffective at the least.

Essential Oils can be an integral part of any healing process, but the person who uses them should be informed as to their proper uses as well as any contraindications. Even the purest, therapeutic grade oils can be used inappropriately.

Therapeutic Essential Oils are known to (w)holistic practitioners as *precious oils* for several reasons:

- Depending on the oil, it can take an entire plant to extract one drop of oil.
- It sometimes requires prodigious amounts of flowers from several plants to create a single drop of oil.
- They are far more potent than dried herbs.
- They can last for millennia; they have been found in the pyramids of Kemet with their integrity intact.
- They are oxygen transporters.
- They do not accumulate in the body.
- They have been successfully used in the healing process of many specific imbalances.
- Appropriately used oils do not have dangerous or negative side effects.

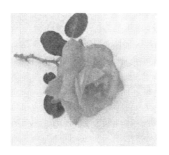

*"Essential Oils are
the missing link..."*
- Dr Gary Young

I use Young Living Essential Oils, because I have researched and found them to be of impeccable quality and efficiency. I did not come to this conclusion lightly, but after visiting one of their farms and distilleries in Utah, (they have over 2,000 acres of organic farmland in the US and in France) witnessing the process from seed to oil, and actually spending time with Dr. and Mrs. Young, I can attest to the high level of integrity of their oils and other supplements. Young Living oils are truly therapeutic, frequently tested, and often *exceed* the standards of testing.

The use of Essential Oils in ancient Kemet is documented on the pyramid walls, as well as in the Ebers Papyrus, a Kemetian medical scroll which dates back to 1500 BC. The same papyrus also shows evidence of the use of herbal prescriptions, reflexology and massage therapy.

The Kemites used herbs as medicine; they did not casually ingest herbal teas every day, as so many of us have become accustomed to today. Essential Oils were also used as medicine, for ritual ceremonies, for making incense, for embalming and to make their perfumes. More on Essential Oils will be discussed later.

Few people think more than two or three times a year; I have made an international reputation for myself by thinking once a week.

- George Bernard Shaw

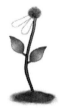

Chapter 3
The First Step
Mindful Living

The Principle of Mentalism

"'THE ALL is MIND; the Universe is Mental'... This principle embodies the truth that 'All is Mind.' It explains that THE ALL (which is the Substantial Reality underlying all the outward manifestations and appearances which we know under the terms of 'The Material Universe'; 'The Phenomena of Life'; 'Matter'; 'Energy'; and in short, all that is apparent to our material senses) is SPIRIT, which in itself is UNKNOWABLE and UNDEFINABLE, but which may be considered and thought of as AN UNIVERSAL, INFINITE, LIVING MIND."

The Kybalion, p26

If you want to be happy, be.

- Leo Tolstoy

There are 2 aspects of the ancient principle of Mentalism that I'd like to explore, while using the more contemporary nomenclature of Mindful Living. One can be considered as causal, the other as effectual.

Causal: Everything in the physical world had its beginning in the realm of cause. The Merriam-Webster Dictionary defines the word *cause* as "*an agent that brings something about*". Metaphysics is the study of cause. The word metaphysics breaks down to m*eta* = beyond or above, and *physical* = form. Thus, the study of Metaphysics is the study of what is beyond the physical. It is the metaphysical that brings about everything that we see, touch hear, taste and feel.

Thinking is a metaphysical process. Thought is a living force that we can either manipulate, or be manipulated by. In my taped lecture on *The Metaphysics of Health and Healing,* I thoroughly discuss the power and consequences of thought. I also elaborate on the premise that **thought is the genesis of all form**.

Effectual: Mindful Living is an outgrowth (effect) of the first Kemetic principle of Mentalism; it is exercising your ability to live in the present moment. As young children, we were really good at this. Notice how babies are surprised and delighted to see your face each and every time it "appears" in the game of peek-a-boo. Scientists attribute this presence of mind to the underdeveloped state of the infant brain; but, be that as it may (or may not be) they remain in the present. For the infant, every moment is a new one; he doesn't dwell in the past or worry about the future; she simply IS in the moment.

Emancipate yourself
from the past

Think back to when you were a young child. Remember riding in a car for 2 hours with your parents and feeling like you've been riding for 12? ("Are we there yet?") The *now* was all that there was for you; nothing else existed. It was the same for all of us.

Somewhere along the way, we take a detour down an illusory path of time that clouds our consciousness until we can no longer see ourselves *in the moment*. We begin to see our lives only in terms of past or future events.

Consequently we develop a new self-image that draws exclusively on previous experiential agreements and how they may relate to future events. We completely overlook our presence in the now. This new self does not know or remember how to be free as a child is free, so it learns a new way to be.

We learn to attach mounting significance to painful disturbing experiences of the past; we learn to associate, cross-reference and remember every minute detail of our distresses, and use them as the foundational platform for all our future experiences; yes, we become quite proficient in remembering the pain.

This is an unproductive application of the powerful principle of Mentalism that greatly narrows our choices for achieving the positive outcomes of Mindful Living.

You cannot live tomorrow...

Bring yourself back to the present moment

Dwelling on a painful past experience brings that event into the present moment, causing us to re-live the same fear, pain or anger that we originally did. During the time that we spend lamenting and re-living the past, we literally **are reliving** the experience, negatively affecting the *now* in our bodies as well as our spirit-souls and minds.

I remember a young lady who was in the downtown area of New York City on the infamous day of September 11th, in 2001. She managed to escape physical injury as she ran all the way from Manhattan to Brooklyn (approximately 7 miles) without shoes, in shock and fear, but the emotional trauma of what she witnessed with her eyes and her spirit was altogether debilitating.
For at least 2 years, she was unable to talk about that devastating experience without having her legs ache and cramp with real, unimagined pain. It was evident that her muscles held on to the memory of the trauma.

We forfeit the present when reliving the past; we may be using our eyes, but we are not really seeing; we may hear, but we no longer know how to listen.

Our nerves, hormones and inner organs don't know the difference between yesterday and today; they only follow the instructions that we send with our immediate thoughts, feelings and emotions. Our thoughts replay our experiences with the assistance of chemical messengers (neurotransmitters); our feelings and emotions engage to create deeper imprints of the memory of the experience; then our organs, muscles, cells and nerves repeat the same physiological sensations of the past experience, and we in turn relive the pain anew, as in the very first time— *again*.

"Life is thickly sown with thorns, and I know no other remedy than to pass quickly through them. The longer we dwell on our misfortunes, the greater is their power to harm us."

- Voltaire, (1694-1778)

With memory set smarting like a reopened wound, a man's past is not simply a dead history, an outworn preparation of the present: it is not a repented error shaken loose from the life: it is a still quivering part of himself, bringing shudders and bitter flavors and the tinglings of a merited shame.

George Eliot (1819-1880)

This whole process weakens our internal defenses, leaving us ever more vulnerable to imbalances in the spirit-body connection, inevitably leading to dis-ease.

Conversely, releasing and truly forgiving past negative experiences—as well as not worrying about what might happen in the future—allows us to find an enduring, peaceful state of being. I know this is much easier said than done, but it has been done by many, and **can** be done by you through the practice of Mindful Living. You have the same power to choose your experiential agreements as everyone else.[2] Remember:

"The Universe is mental—held in the mind of THE ALL" - The Kybalion

The Kybalion teaches us that there is nothing greater than "Infinite Living Mind"; for that is the substance of "The All".

"The All creates in its Infinite Mind countless Universes, which exist for eons of time—and yet, to THE ALL, the creation, development, decline and death of a million Universes is of the time of the twinkling of an eye" -The Kybalion

---

[2] Read *The Master Mind by* Theron Dumont

We all know the old expression "Time waits for no man"; that's only partially true. When we chose to appreciate the present moment more, worry about the future less, and observe the power of Infinite Mind working within our own minds, time no longer has relevance.

Being Mindful of the present does not mean neglecting the future. We all have plans, goals and aspirations that are fueled by our intentions. The future has a definite place in the mind of the Mindful Being. That place is one of hope—not of worry and fear; it's a place of encouragement and precise, determined planning with tangible expectations.

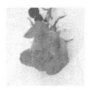

"*Things without remedy should be without regard; what is done is done.*"

- William Shakespeare (1564-1616)

Mindful Living Exercises

1. Just for one day, purposefully observe and focus on every detail that you can. Look around the room when you wake up; notice smells, sounds and colors; try not to judge or evaluate, just observe. Shower or bathe with your full, undivided attention on every detail of the experience.

2. Listen carefully to your own thoughts throughout the day. Really listen to others when engaged in conversation. Listen with your eyes as well as with your ears; listen to their intent as well as the content of their communication, and listen without thinking of what you will say in response. (That's a "toughie"☺)

3a. Try eating your meals without being distracted by talk-radio or TV. Observe food on your plate as though seeing it for the first time; appreciate the effort that was made to produce it; offer thanks to whomever or whatever you will.

Consider the soil and rain, the sun and the seasons that were in agreement with the creation of what you have on your plate; slowly chew and savor each morsel in your mouth. How does it feel? How does it taste? Follow it down your throat to your stomach. Notice how you feel before, during and after eating.

b) Do not eat when you are angry or upset. When you do, your food becomes partially indigestible and toxic, due to a chemical reaction to your emotional distress. In the art of Mindful Living, it's better to wait until you internally resolve your conflicts, have a few sips of water, take a few deep breaths, and *then* enjoy your meal in peace.

c) Choose a specific time to devote to your dreams and goals every day. Write them down; get pictures, and while you're planning, experience them in the present moment. Then return your focus to the activities of the day.

"What luck for rulers that men do not think!"

Adolph Hitler

Essential Oil Recommendations

(According to the Essential Oil Desk Reference)[3]

Present Time: A blend of Neroli, Ylang Ylang, and Spruce.
It is an empowering fragrance that creates a feeling of being in the moment.

Angelica (angelica archangelica) is used to assist in the releasing of pent-up, negative feelings.

EO's Used for Agitation

Single: Bergamot, cedarwood, clary sage, frankincense, geranium, juniper, lavender, myrrh, marjoram, rosewood, rose, ylang ylang, sandalwood.

Blends: Peace & Calming, Joy, Valor, Harmony, Forgiveness, Chivalry.

---

[3] Third Edition, Essential Science Publishing

Essential Oils used for anxiety

Single: Orange, Roman Chamomile, tangerine, Ylang Ylang, Lavender, Frankincense

Blends: Valor, Hope, Peace & Calming, Present Time, Joy, Citrus Fresh, Surrender, Believe.

EO's Used for Concentration

Single: Cedarwood, cypress, juniper, lavender, lemon, basil, helichrysum, myrrh, orange, peppermint, rosemary, sandalwood, ylang ylang.

Blends: Clarity, Awaken, Gathering, Dream Catcher, Magnify Your Purpose, Brain Power.

"Sometimes I think and other times I am."

Paul Valéry, 1924
Variété: Cantiques spirituels,

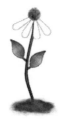

Chapter 4

The Second Step
Agreement

The Principle of Correspondence

"This Principle embodies the truth that there is always a Correspondence between the laws and phenomena of the various planes of Being and Life. The old Hermetic axiom ran in these words: 'As above, so below; as below so above.'"

– The Kybalion, p28

OUR SECOND STEP OF AGREEMENT RELATES TO the second principle of Correspondence in that whatever you agree to with your mind, you will reflect in the actions of your body. We have a way of separating our lives into isolated units that (we believe) are totally unrelated to each other.

"My people and I have come to an agreement which satisfied us both. They are to say what they please, and I am to do what I please."

- Frederick the Great

Neat (or not so neat) mental categories of separation help us to rationalize and justify our thoughts, actions and the world. But in reality everything we think, say and do is connected to something else.

When you first heard or saw the title of this book, did you expect to read about metaphysical principles? Did you expect nutritional advice? Or were you simply curious? Perhaps you were completely without expectation. Your expectations stem from your own personal agreements of perception. From *my* personal experiences, I have come to agree that **health is the complete expression of one's innermost balance, peace and strength.**

Healing is the returning of all aspects of the self to the space from which health originally emanates. There is never a time when you don't have an expression of health; there are occasions however, when you reflect a response to unfavorable internal occurrences, but this too is health being expressed.

For some of us, a discussion about health is only about *diet* in the form of what to eat or not to eat. For others it's just about not being sick, or being free of pain. We each hold our own perception of what constitutes health, but if we consider the above definition of health we can see how the 7

Steps and the Kybalion go hand-in-hand toward its fulfillment.

By writing, I have agreed to share 7 Principles of Healing, and by reading you have agreed to at least take a long enough look to see if these pages hold anything else that you can accept, learn from, agree or disagree with.

Whatever you fully agree with will remain with you until it becomes an integral part of you. It will remain an integral part of you until you consciously change your agreement, just as you have always done since before you can even remember. If or when you agree to change or release that agreement, you will do so by replacing it with another one, and so you will continue along in your personal journey.

"Health nuts are going to feel stupid someday, lying in hospitals dying of nothing."

- Redd Foxx

Let the law of Correspondence remind you that you are a reflection of the Universe. "As above, so below, as below, so above" The Universe is reflected within you.

The earth is 30% landmass, and 70% water; in reflective agreement you are 30% tissue-matter, and 70% fluid. There are infinite possibilities in the Universe, and infinite possibilities are within you. "As above, so below".

Dr. Deepak Chopra expresses this aspect of your existence in his book *Live Longer, Grow Younger* when he states

"If you are able to look at yourself as a field of possibilities, intimately interrelated to everything else, wonderful new opportunities develop."[4]

Your present existence is manifested in a consciousness paradigm that is cosmically calibrated by your thoughts. In the context of healing and wellbeing, remember that the manner in which you sustain your physical body is consciously or unconsciously a creation of your thoughts, which lead to actions generated by the chemicals, enzymes, hormones and electrical signals that send messages throughout your entire being.

---

[4] See *Live Longer, Grow Younger* by Deepak Chopra MD and David Simon, MD p12.

In agreement with the power of your mind (thoughts), you can create whatever you decide to. Subconsciously, you do it all the time. You create appetites, and you create moods; both of which create the environment that is a reflection of yourself.

Moods can be created in us by thoughts, scents, visual stimulation and music, as well as by emotional feelings. Appetites are not only created by the taste buds on our tongues, or the sensation of fullness in the belly; they are also developed by and *through the emotional feelings we connect to physical feelings of satiation.* Those emotional feelings are again reinforced by our subconscious thoughts and Agreements.

Through habit, we develop appetites for food, music, activities, and just about anything we can imagine. We can even develop an appetite for certain moods. Moods, like thought, can take on their own consciousness, and like children, demand that you nurture them with your attention. Through the use of conscious thought, we can chose to focus more on, and realize more of the infinite possibilities which Deepak Chopra speaks of, and purposefully create the habits, moods and appetites that will keep us in Agreement with good health.

Agreement

In his teachings, metaphysician Dr. Phillip Valentine speaks of "particle perception". He is referring to infinitesimal photonic particles that are extracted from light-waves as they are called upon by human perception.

Through intent (the prelude to thought), you gather these intangible particles from the cosmic spectrum as a magnet would little shavings of metal, except *these* particles consist of photons of light. They are not scattered, bunched or chaotic; they are ordered by Divine Intelligence and directed by Human Intent. These particles that constitute perception become the photonic medium by which you communicate throughout your entire being at the speed of thought—which is faster than that of light. Actually, it is thought that directs the light.

Your thoughts direct the light as you create your own unique reality...

You are a creator. There is nothing new under or beyond the sun, yet you still create your own unique conglomeration of photonic particles, and mold them into moods, situations and eventually into the templates that become the *physical* manifestations of your conscious and unconscious agreements. The agreements we create today will remain in the ether, serve their purpose, run their course, and continue to be a self-fulfilling prophesy, unless and until we change the metaphysical template.

Even when you are not aware of what you are doing, you are creating. The simple example of what happens when you cut yourself on the finger proves this truth. Without assistance from anyone or anything, you create the necessary cells and tissues to repair the wound and heal; you bleed to clean the area; the injured tissue cells release histamine and other chemicals, while plasma, white blood cells and antibodies flood the area; specified proteins create fibrin which helps form a blood-clot; the clot holds the edges of the wound together, and isolates the area to prevent harmful substances from spreading to the rest of your body; new capillaries and other blood vessels form to bring blood and nutrients to the area. You then begin creating new skin (granulated tissue) that will eventually be replaced by permanent skin.

"The world we have created is a product of our thinking; it cannot be changed without changing our thinking."

— Albert Einstein

Without assistance from anyone or anything, you unconsciously create and assemble the essential components for healing. This is your personal agreement with the movement of Cosmic Intelligence of the Most High.

As mentioned before, most of the time we are not intentionally and purposefully creating; but conscious realization and complete innerstanding of this fact makes it possible for us to heal ourselves "at will" with the use of focused intention.

"What we call reality is an agreement that people have arrived at to make life more livable"

- Louise Nevelson 1900 - 1988

Agreement

In his book of Toltec wisdom entitled *The Four Agreements*, Don Miguel Ruiz reveals the simple truth that everything we believe, accept and do is based on the agreements we hold. Therefore at any given moment, by making a decision we can change our agreements, and thus manipulate reality. The key is to be honest enough with ourselves to acknowledge the agreements that we have placed on "automatic pilot". These are the unconscious agreements that cause us to think the same thoughts and make the same judgments and decisions, even when we don't want to. They are also the agreements that help us to convince and reassure ourselves that we are "right" or "justified" in thinking those thoughts, making those judgments, etc....

Again, by consciously choosing your agreements, you have the ability to create anything you decide to.

You will always have a choice.

The significant problems we face cannot be solved at the same level of thinking we were at when we created them."

— Albert Einstein

The Bhagavad-Gita, an ancient Dravidian text written more than 150 thousand years ago states:

"When thou shalt rise beyond the plane of illusion, then shalt thou cease to disturb thyself regarding doctrines, theology, disputations concerning rites or ceremonies, and other useless trimmings upon the cloth of spiritual thought."

The phrase "cease to disturb thyself" can be particularly helpful in times of stress. It can bring clarity and comfort by reminding you that you don't have to "agree" to be caught-up in an emotional state of frustration—if you choose not to. The text continues:

"You will be liberated from those who would interpret that which they fail themselves to understand; but instead, shalt thou fix thy mind in earnest contemplation of the spirit, and thus reach the harmony of thy true self" (ibid)

In more contemporary jargon we would say "Free your mind of the dictates of others. Envision your goal; know what you want, and go for it. Be at peace with yourself."

When you are ready, you will decide to intentionally spend more time with your Divine Self. You will choose to promote the conscious and unconscious agreements that invariably lead to the expression of good health; you will agree to choose, appreciate, enjoy and eventually *prefer* foods that strengthen instead of weaken you; you will no longer agree that you can't find the time to start and *stay* on a sensible exercise plan; you will agree to eventually connect with others that are on the same path; they will appreciate the same things, and seek the same health benefits that you do. And finally, you will no longer agree to judge yourself or anyone else.

Granted, this is all much easier said than done, but when you fall short of your goals, you'll simply start again, following *your own path* to health and wellbeing—not someone else's. The issue of judgment here is a very important one, because judgment is an agreement of "temporary finality". In other words, based on your own consciousness developments you may find your judgments of yesterday no longer valid today as you agree to no longer judge. For the dedicated seeker, there really is no need or place for judgment. She/He realizes (for instance) that what we eat, do or choose as our life style can improve our expression of health, but it cannot make us "better" people. If others choose to eat, be or do x, y or z, so be it, it's their choice. Their choices are just that—*their* choices, their agreements, and nothing more.

When you are in agreement with your Higher Self, your spirit will more often rise to re-visit your space of contentment, until you eventually remain in that peaceful state. Your physical body will reflect this agreement with improved health and increased vitality.

Please note that my use of the term "higher self" does not mean "better self" in terms of good or bad. "Higher" refers to the velocity and frequency plane of your vibrations; the higher the velocity, the lighter and subtler the vibration will be.

In your true "self" there is no density or weight, except as it is manifested as a quality through the emotions that connect the choices, judgments or agreements that you make.

Your higher self is the part of you that constitutes the core essence of your being. It is that aspect of consciousness that contains the blueprint of all healing. It is the Breath of Life that permeates and flows in your CranioSacral Fluid. It is the child of Cosmic Intelligence— just one aspect of the One Most High—fostered and focused by Infinite Intent.

Judgment is the precursor to the emotional weight that becomes the initiator of all forms of stress, eventually leading to dis-ease.

Whatever you do, you need courage. Whatever course you decide upon, there is always someone to tell you that you are wrong. There are always difficulties arising that tempt you to believe your critics are right. To map out a course of action and follow it to an end requires some of the same courage that a soldier needs. Peace has its victories, but it takes brave men and women to win them.

- Ralph Waldo Emerson *(1803-1882)*

"Things without remedy should be without regard; what is done is done."

\- William Shakespeare *(1564-1616)*

Agreement Cognizance Exercise

1. Write down on paper 3 new agreements that you would like to make regarding yourself and the rest of the Universe. These will be the opposite of certain agreements that you may have had all of your life before now.

2. Then write 3 statements that confirm each of your new agreements. (That will make 9 in all) For example, if you've had trouble with math you can say: "I'm better at math than I used to be; I like dealing with numbers. Every day, I find it easier to do math calculations.

3. In the evening before you go to bed, and every morning as soon as you awake, repeat the 3 statements of one of your new agreements, for a minimum of 21 days without interruption. If you find that you still don't believe your statements, give yourself an additional 21 days of affirmations.

4. Repeat the process with your other 2 new agreements.

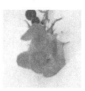

Essential Oil Recommendations

Patchouli (Pogostemon cablin)

- is often used to assist in the release of insecurity, jealousy and obsessive thoughts.

Spruce (Picea Mariana)

- Releases emotional blocks.
The Lakota Natives used Spruce to strengthen their ability to communicate with the Great Spirit.

Essential Oil Recommendations

Valor©
- a proprietary blend of Rosewood, Blue Tansy, Frankincense and Spruce

- Balances energies to instill courage, confidence and self esteem. It helps the body self-correct its balance and alignment

White Angelica
- a proprietary blend of Ylang Ylang, Rose, Melissa, Sandalwood, Geranium, Spruce, Myrrh, Hyssop, Bergamot and Rosewood

- Increases the aura around the body, and helps create a realization of wholeness; it neutralizes negative energy.

Essential Oil Recommendations

Highest Potential
- a proprietary blend of Austrian Blue, Galbanum, Frankincense, Sandalwood, Rose, Lavender, Cinnamon Bark, Spruce, Ylang Ylang, Jasmine Absolute and Geranium

- Harmonizes several grounding, calming inspiring and empowering oils that uplift the spirit, relieve frustration and anger, assist creativity, and clear the thought process.

*As you vibrate, so you
will resonate*

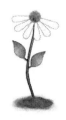

Chapter 5
The Third Step

Resonance

The Principle of Vibration

"This principle embodies the truth that 'everything is in motion'; everything vibrates'; nothing is at rest'; facts which Modern Science endorses, and which each new scientific discovery tends to verify."

- The Kybalion, p30

THE STANDARD COLLEGE DICTIONARY DEFINES resonance as: "the property whereby any vibratory system responds with maximum amplitude to an applied force having a frequency equal or nearly equal to its own."

*Vibration is to resonance as intent
is to thought*

You are a vibratory system. When you respond (and sometimes retort) to a comment, gesture or even a look from another individual, you are resonating with their pre-determined level of vibrational frequency.

Everything vibrates—Trees, plants, flowers, animals, rocks, humans—everything. Depending upon our state of emotional or physical health, we vibrate in higher faster frequencies of vibrations, or lower slower ones at any given time. Different "parts" of our being (brain, organs, etc.) also vibrate at different rates, according to their necessary functions.

Although everything vibrates, everything does not necessarily resonate in similar spaces of harmonic synchronicity. To resonate, a given entity must either meet other matching vibrations, or reverberate (bounce off of another entity), and return to meet itself at the same amplitude.

Your pre-existing perceptions, assumptions and beliefs are nurtured and formed by your intent into a conclusive thought. Each thought carries its own unique wave-patterns of vibration—also governed by your intent. In the same fashion, your level of vibration will determine how you will resonate.

"The molecular arrangement of the physical body is actually a complex network of interwoven energy fields"

- *Vibrational Medicine*
Dr Richard Gerber, MD

When you meet someone for the first time and immediately feel as though you've known each other already, it's partially because at that moment you both are sending vibrations that are reflecting, echoing, reverberating and returning to each of you respectively, and at the same amplitude; you are both resonating.

The ancient spiritual guides knew the importance of understanding the principle of vibration, and shared it with us as the third Kemetic law of the Kybalion. Today we have scientific instruments that can measure the frequencies of vibration, for those who need visual scientific "proof".

The vibrations of humans, food, plants, etc., can be measured in Hertz (Hz).[5]

Dr. Gary Young, naturopath and world-renowned essential oil specialist, conducted a test with more than 200 subjects at Eastern State University in Washington. He wanted to ascertain and document the effects of certain food substances and essential oils on the vibration frequencies of the human body.

Dr. Young noted that the average body frequency ranged from 62 to 68Hz. Brain frequencies are

---

[5]   Hertz was one of the scientists of the early eighteenth century, who benefited from the pillaging of ancient scientific records of electronics by Napoleon from Kemet.

10Hz higher than the body during the day, and 10Hz lower at night. When you are well, you are vibrating on the frequency of 66 to 70Hz. When you are vibrating at 58Hz, you are not feeling well. This is where—due to cellular electromagnetic imbalances—dis-ease can begin:

If we throw Mother Nature out the window, she comes back in the door with a pitchfork."

-Masanobu Fukuoka

"...Flu starts at 57(Hz) Candida at 55; Epstein-Barr at 52 and Cancer at 42."[6]

In one of those tests at the University two healthy young men, each with at 66H frequency, were tested. One was given a cup of coffee to hold in his hand; in 3 seconds his vibrational frequency dropped to 58 Hz. The other was given a cup of coffee to drink, and after drinking, his vibrations dropped to 52Hz; he was not given an essential oil to inhale, and it took 3 days for his vibration frequency to return to 66Hz.

Thought, light, music, food, color, emotions, and the quality of air that you breathe can affect your frequency level of vibrations. Therapeutic Grade Essential Oils have the ability to assist in raising your vibrations and facilitate healing. This cannot necessarily be done with oils you may find at your health food store, because they are either cut with chemicals (i.e. propylene glycol) processed quickly, and/or at high temperatures.

In the U.S. these oils can be processed with all of the above, and be sold as "100% pure essential oils". They may smell really good as they carry the same scents, but they do not resonate at

---

[6] Dr Gary Young. The Missing Link Audio book, ©2000

therapeutic grade levels. Most truly therapeutic grade Essential Oils can be ingested[7].

"Quantum physics has found that there is no empty space in the human cell, but it is a teeming, electric-magnetic field of possibility or potential" -Dr. D. Chopra

---

[7]Essential oils should only be used with the guidance of a health care professional.

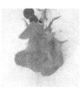

Essential Oil Recommendations

Neroli Absolute (Citrus Aurantium)

Highly regarded by the Ancient Kemites for its
ability to raise vibrations, and heal body, mind
and spirit

Orange (Citrus Sinensis)

- Anti-tumoral, antidepressant, assists
defense system, emotionally uplifting

"On such things as matter we have all been wrong, what we have called matter is energy, whose vibration has been so lowered as to be perceptible to the senses. There is no matter."

-Albert Einstein

Although some companies are beginning to claim that their oils are therapeutic, they don't meet the standard[8]. Only 2% of Essential Oils processed in the U.S. vibrate at therapeutic grade levels. The terms "natural", "pure" and "organic" do not necessarily mean that they retain the resonant quality of therapeutic grade oils.[9]

Flower Essences can also affect your resonance capacity. **Bach Flower Remedies** created by Dr. Edward Bach, are homeopathic tinctures of particular flower blends used to therapeutically raise one's resonance quotient. Dr. Bach was a bacteriologist and homeopathic physician in the early 20th century. In 1930 he realized that the subtle energies of certain essences matched the vibrations of the human subtle body. When humans are emotionally off balance, (therefore vibrating on lower hertz frequencies) Bach Flower essences can be used to help bring relief. They are highly recommended in emergency situations, and post traumatic recovery (from near fatal accidents and the sudden loss of a loved one, to trips to the dentist and new job jitters, etc.)

Note: Although these essences are not toxic and have no side effects, one should not make a habit of using them.

---

[8]In the US, a company can use 10% of an essential oil, and claim that it is 100% pure.

[9] To learn more about, or purchase therapeutic essential oils, go to www.healbytouch.com.

Live foods will raise your vibrations

The following are a few items that will enhance your ability to resonate (in) good health:

Food Choices

When food is eaten in its natural state, it will provide the atomic energy necessary for higher, more rapid vibrations. Food grown in soil that hasn't been sprayed with noxious chemicals and/or artificial fertilizers in 4 to 7 years is considered organically grown food. If you choose organic over non-organic foods, you are taking a step towards resonating in/on a higher frequency plane. Sprayed and processed foods on the other hand have lower vibrations, will also lower *your* vibrations and weaken your internal defenses.

The closer the food is to its natural state, the more your body will recognize it, and the less metabolic enzymes, and life-force (energy, qi) you will have to expend to process it.

By choosing to buy organic products, you support the organic farmers who are trying to preserve the natural inherent value of the soil and their crops. You also participate in the renewal of the earth for our descendants. Organic farming restores the natural balance of vitamins, minerals and helpful insects to the earth.

As one verse of the Christian Bible says *"My people are destroyed for lack of knowledge..."*[10]

In the western world, we are currently experiencing a serious and insidious health crisis fueled by increasing ignorance, and profited by the food and medical industries and the pharmaceutical companies.

Hypertension, arthritis, obesity and diabetes are rampant; heart disease kills more women than breast cancer, and breast cancer is now appearing in women as young as 17 years of age! As if that weren't horrendous enough, cancer kills more children than any other disease; over 8.5 million children have asthma, *children as young as 3 years of age have fatty deposits in their arteries, and by the time they reach 12, they have the beginning stages of hardening of the arteries!!* Is this not insane?!![11]

People, we were *not* created to live and die this way. We are *not* vibrating in or resonating wellness, we are *not* giving our children the legacy of vibrant health that should be their birthright, and we are *not* living to *at least* the age of 120 as our cells and DNA should be well equipped to carry us to! The ironic truth is that *every one* of

---

[10] Hosea 4:6

[11] Watch for my book on healthy children

those so-called "degenerative diseases" is preventable. Prevention is the key.

Since there is no such thing as a cure, Prevention is without a doubt, the best approach to healing

"Intellectuals solve problems; geniuses prevent them"

- Albert Einstein 1879-1955

To remind ourselves of what true health looks and feels like, we need only to return to the simple, basic, daily incorporation of healthy food choices, non-stressful thought patterns and lifestyles, regular, sensible exercise and copious amounts of pure water. Granted, our society has made it more difficult, but it certainly is possible to do all these to maintain wellness, and prevent illnesses; we only need to *set our intent to do so.*

As I mentioned before, fresh, raw, organic fruits and vegetables have the atomic energy we need to keep our internal vibrations high, and to resonate with true wellness. This is mainly due to the enzyme activity these foods assist our bodies with. You see, we create different enzymes for different bodily functions that keep us alive. *Enzymes are imperative for life itself.*

In his book *Enzyme Nutrition, the Food Enzyme Concept,* Dr. Edward Howell explains how these vital enzymes function in our bodies.

"To get enzymes from food, one must eat raw food. All life, whether plant or animal, requires the presence of enzymes to keep it going...The mere touch of heat destroys them"[12]

---

[12] Enzyme Nutrition, p 5

Without enzymes, food is literally dead. Dr. Howell proved that when we eat lifeless, cooked food, our body has to make up for the deficit of food enzymes by creating more dietary enzymes. This is done at the expense of metabolic enzymes needed to perform other functions for our organs.

You can see why I continue to repeat "We must eat lots of fresh, raw fruits and vegetables". It is recommended by the US government that we eat an average of 10 servings of organic produce every day, to assist our bodies in counter-acting environmental stress, as well as protecting and repairing our cellular DNA. The conundrum is that most of us either can't, don't or won't get all that produce in a week—not to mention a day! (Is it any wonder we don't live to be 140 years old like the Hunza people do?)

When I was diagnosed with breast cancer in 1996, surgery was the only option offered to me by doctors of the medical profession. I chose not to take that option but instead, to seek a natural approach to healing.[13] It may sound brave, but I was scared to death! After all, when your doctor pronounces the "cancer sentence", you think of all the discouraging statistics on cancer, and you just *know* you're facing death. No, I was not

---

[13] This was my own personal experience, and is not meant as a suggestion for anyone else.

brave; I just knew what didn't want—surgery, radiation or chemotherapy!

I was put on a program based on the healing principles of Hygienic Science (These principles were founded on the life-philosophies of the ancient Kemites, and resurrected in the 1800's by Dr. Isaac Jennings, Dr. Russell T. Trall, Dr. Herbert Shelton and other medical doctors.)

Juicing raw, organic fruits and vegetables was a major part of my healing process. At that time, I didn't realize there was another way to get that much whole-food nutrition into my blood-stream to assist in my healing. Since then, I've learned about *Juice Plus+* and found out that it is the nutrition of 15 raw fruits and vegetables and the fiber of 2 grains in a capsule, using the best possible way to preserve enzymes in raw foods— slow dehydration.[14]

Make no mistake: *There is no better nourishment than fresh out-of–the-garden, raw, organic fruits and vegetables!* But as I said before, most of us (even we Vegans) either don't get the *variety,* or we don't get the *quantity* raw foods to protect our DNA from the constant barrage of free radical damage that we face daily, and Juice Plus+ is the

---

[14] To learn more about Juice Plus+, go to jpnalani.com

next best thing to insure the quantity, as well as the variety of raw produce and enzymes we need.

I don't even consider Juice Plus+ as a supplement; it is the juice of those 15 fruits, vegetables (separate from each other), dehydrated with the sugar removed and 2 grains. That's it. Food—not isolated vitamins.

"While we may not be able to control all that happens to us, we can control what happens inside us."

- Benjamin Franklin

Speaking of Vitamins

Although they are a trillion dollar industry, vitamins have not impacted the world health crisis one iota.

Vitamins *in the body* are really enzymes (which are by the way, proteins internally created by all living organisms that function as catalysts). In other words, we can create certain vitamins as needed. Remember, I said the body recognizes *foods*. I should have said it recognizes "whole" foods. "Whole foods" are foods that have all of their vitamins, minerals and other enzymes intact, and in proper proportions. Our bodies know exactly how to utilize whole foods.

Scientists have isolated *10,000* of possibly *12,000 (or more)* constituents of individual fruits and vegetables!

When a vitamin is singularly extracted from food and introduced into the body it (the body) has to make adjustments to compensate for the other missing ingredients of that food. Consequently, a number of reactions can be expected:

First of all, the body will not recognize it as food, but will respond as it does to drugs (herbs included). To reiterate, this is not to say that vitamins, herbs and other supplements should never be used— there is a time and place for almost everything—but it *is* to say that we cannot expect our bodies to function with artificial compounds as they would with the "real thing."

If you have a deficiency and think you may need nutritional supplementation, it's best to deal with supplements that are more like whole foods, with the intention of re-balancing yourself to the place where you will no longer need supplements. You don't have an isolated vitamin deficiency; you have a whole food deficiency. You should also consult with a nutritionist that understands this ortho-biotic truth; unfortunately, not all do.

"If all the medicine in the world were thrown into the sea, it would be bad for the fish and good for humanity"

-         O.W. Holmes,
(Prof. of Med. Harvard University)

Sometimes when taking supplements, we get an initial positive reaction because the body has been "tricked" into functioning as though it has what it needs. Meanwhile the *cause* of the imbalance is not being addressed. It may appear that one is benefiting from the vitamin, but eventually the organ(s) that had to process the vitamin—as an unnatural substance—will begin to show signs of stress. This scenario is compounded when herbs are introduced into the body. Prolonged use of herbs could foster a dependency, and could also be potentially damaging to the liver and kidneys.

Research reported in *the Journal of the American Medical Association* and other sources indicates that isolated Vitamin E actually increases the risk of heart disease. Antioxidant vitamins like A, D and E can be harmful when taken regularly and in large dosages, because unlike vitamin C which the body cannot produce or store, but uses immediately discarding the excess, vitamins A, D and E *are* stored in the body and can be over-dosed.

Vitamin D that is made by the skin utilizing the direct resonant rays of the sun is more readily metabolized that an artificial, chemical vitamin D analog. In fact, researchers have found vitamin D supplements to be totally ineffective in numerous studies. The best way to get sufficient vitamin D is to get direct sunlight without wearing glasses of any type. If you don't get out often but intend to increase your exposure to the sun it is *imperative* that you do so gradually. This is a major key to sun safety.

The more melanin you have, the more direct sunlight you require to synthesize vitamin D. Melanin absorbs and utilizes the ultra-violet rays, lowering the levels of D in the bloodstream.

I would also be very wary of using sun blocks. Chemically loaded sun blocking lotions and creams are supposed to protect from the sun, but they actually have been linked to skin cancer.[15]

---

[15]See internet articles "Sun Blocks Can Actually Increase Your Cancer Risk" by Dr Joseph Mercola, and "Sunlight for Your Life" by Dr. Jamie Fattig,

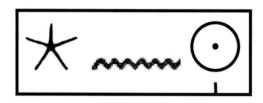

"Dwa n Ra"

Thanks for the Sun

"*What sunshine is to flowers, smiles are to humanity. These are but trifles, to be sure; but scattered along life's pathway, the good they do is inconceivable.*"

\- Joseph Addison

More on Fruits and vegetables

To reiterate, raw, organic fruits and vegetables, each containing their own unique forms of nutritive water, have higher resonant vibrations than meat and starchy foods like white bread and pasta, which are dead, with little or no nutritionally resonant energizing life-force, because they are closer to their original state. In their natural condition, live foods offer the more complete spectrum of nutrition, including their easily assimilated juices and higher levels of atomic energy. In addition to the vital enzymes discussed before, the juices of raw fruits and vegetables also have alkalizing properties that help to neutralize blood toxins. Remember, the closer your food is to being in its natural state, the more nutritious it will be.

As they grow and ripen in the sun, fruits and vegetables not only soak in pure, radiant energy, but they synthesize those rays into phytonutrients[16], many of which are actually the pigmentation that give the fruit or vegetable its color. Color is the reflection of photonic particles. It is light-energy encapsulated in various photonic wavelength measurements; it is the visibility of the electromagnetic spectrum of light, as it resonates with photon receptors of the eyes.

---

[16] Phyto=plant.

Remember the saying "The darker the berry, the sweeter the juice"? The same can be said regarding vibration frequencies of fruits and vegetables: The riper the fruit, the higher the vibration will be (but not when it's over-ripe).

By-the-way, fruits and vegetables are meant to ripen on the vine. When produce is picked early, before ripening, green and hard, (as it's done to get them to the stores with little spoilage and damage) it is missing the additional nutrients it would have received in the last few days on the vine. It will get softer as it sits on your window sill, but it will not ripen.

Now don't be discouraged if you live in an apartment, and/or do not have space for a garden. There are several things you can do to keep your vibrations high with organic fruits and vegetables:

- Shop at Farmer's Markets in your area
- Buy organic whenever you can.
- Grow vegetables on your windowsill (I did, it's fun☺)
- Grow them in large planters on the floor near a window
- Get a juicer
- Take your Juice Plus+
- When dining out, choose restaurants that prepare organic foods.

"The news isn't that fruits and vegetables are good for you; it's that they are so good for you they could save your life"[17]

-   TIME Magazine, Oct. 2003

---

[17] This may be news for the medical community, but naturopaths have been teaching this "news" for at least 150 years.

The darker the fruit the more carotinoids and melanin contained therein, therefore the more solar-based nutrients it will have. Fresh, raw produce is loaded with nutritious enzymatic activity; when you eat it your body more readily recognizes and receives its nutrients, and consequently, you resonate in a higher frequency of vibration.

Another gift of the sun is the more subtle atomic energy that I spoke of earlier. Dr. David Cousens M.D. devotes a considerable portion of his book *Conscious Eating* to the energetic nature of food. In it, he speaks of Subtle Organizing Energy Fields (SOEF's) as energy patterns that all living entities are surrounded and permeated by. Cousens writes:

"A nutrient in this context is what we absorb into our overall body-mind-spirit from the different density levels that have precipitated from the cosmic force. Material food is the densest; sunlight is the least dense on the material plane, and the pure cosmic energy is the most subtle nutrient."[18]

If we can be more cognizant of the more subtle, higher vibrational aspect of our existence, we will find it considerably easier to make the choices that will nourish, enhance and extend the

---

[18] See *Conscious Eating* Pg 275.

duration of our experience in this consciousness paradigm.

A table, a chair, a bowl of fruit and a violin; what else does a man need to be happy?"

- Albert Einstein

Drinking Water

If you have a kidney disorder, or you find that you are not releasing as much water as you are drinking, speak with your doctor to ascertain how much water you should (or should not) be drinking.

Before we discuss the crucial necessity of water as a maintainer of life, human health and well being, I would like to interject our conversation here with a statement about the increasingly controversial question of distilled vs. non-distilled water.

There are very convincing and persuasive arguments against the use of distilled water that are based on scientific research. This research appears on the surface to be valid and conclusive, but if one is willing (or able) to look at the question with a truly wholistic eye, one would see that the scientific research on distilled water remains inconclusive, and tends to misconstrue certain intrinsic actions of the human cell based on Divine Intelligence—for example, its innate ability to use whatever is available towards improving its state of existence—as a negative reaction to the drinking of distilled water.

Re-acquaint your deeper cellular network with the awesome power of water, and resonate with good health

Remember, medical science uses the observation and categorization of effects, not the *intrinsic* dynamics of cause.

Distilled or "soft" water has had ALL impurities removed from it, including the minerals you would otherwise find in it. As a result, it can have a "magnetic" effect on what it interfaces with. When we drink distilled water, our bodies use it to assist in the continuous process of cellular purification more aggressively than it does with non-distilled, mineralized, or "hard" water.

The assumption on the part of researchers is that since excess minerals are eliminated along with toxic cellular waste, the body is losing vital nutrients; they don't consider that those minerals could be in excess, because they are functioning from a premise based on a predetermined paradigm of what constitutes health; again, dismissing any consideration of innate cellular intelligence, as well as failing to overstand the real sources of cellular nutrition (the sun and the chemical gases of the ether). Your body does not discard what is vital for its existence.

I drink distilled water, and have for 25 years; I do not have any of the reported ill effects; my bone density is solid (pun intended), my blood is alkaline, and I have no negative kidney, heart or cardiovascular symptoms whatsoever. I know of others who have used distilled water as their only source of water for longer than 35 years, with the same results.

To distill or not to distill will be debated for many more years to come, until conclusive evidence based on a wholistic premise is well known. Regardless as to what water you choose to drink, know that your body needs copious amounts of it to function properly. Whether you drink distilled, filtered or purified water (as I do all three), you will receive the many benefits of this most important element. Water is so vital for your existence, that you could even drink (dare I say it?) tap water (YECH!) and still get life-saving benefits from it. Bear in mind that tap water is loaded with contaminants, and even toxic waste; it's definitely NOT the water of choice!

Dr. F. Batmanghelidj, MD is probably the most authoritative and knowledgeable person on the subject of drinking water. His book *"Your Body's Many Cries for Water"* is one of the most important books you could ever read. In it, Dr. Batmanghelidj explains and documents how many serious, so-called diseases that are commonly treated with medicines are in reality the consequences of chronic cellular dehydration.

"Chronic cellular dehydration painfully and prematurely kills. Its initial outward manifestations have until now been labeled as diseases of unknown origin"

-   Dr. F. Batmanghelidj, MD

The fact that drinking high levels of water can significantly reduce the risk of heart disease was confirmed by researchers at Loma Linda University, whose research was reported in the American Journal of Epidemiology.[19] This study proves that drinking high amounts of plain water is as important as exercise, diet, or not smoking in the prevention of coronary heart dis-ease.

Most people know that lots of water is needed to flush waste (cellular waste, toxins, etc.) out of the body. What is not widely known, are the many other functions of water in the body. To gain a full understanding of our need for water, be sure to read *"Your Body's Many Cries for Water"*

The "average" person should be drinking at least one half her/his weight in ounces of water, to assist in a quest to resonate vibrant health— that's a lot of water! You see, as Dr. Batmanghelidj explains it, our bodies are operating with a serious deficit of water; we are dehydrated, and have lost our true sense of thirst. This being the case, we've become accustomed to extracting water out of our cells to be used where necessary. If after functioning in this dysfunctional manner for so long you begin drinking lot's more water, you will find yourself running to eliminate it often, because you are still

---

[19] (Vol. 155, No. 9)

extracting some of it from your cells for metabolic use. In time, the intelligence of your body will cause an adjustment, and you shouldn't have to urinate quite as much—but you will go often. As with every change we ask our bodies to reflect, we must be patient, and give them time.

Remember, you are an electro-magnetic vibrating system, and water is an extremely efficient conductor of electricity.

"The brain uses electrical energy that is generated by the water drive of the energy-generating pumps. With dehydration, the level of energy generation in the brain is decreased .Many functions of the brain that depend on this type of energy become inefficient..."[20]

So give your body what it requires for optimum "brain to cellular systems interface", to raise your vibrations and resonate with a higher expression of health and overall well being.

---

[20] *Your Body's Many Cries for Water,* p56 Dr. Batmanghelidj

"If only a small fraction of what is already known about the effects of sugar were to be revealed in relation to any other material used as a food additive, that material would promptly be banned."

- John Yudkin MD, Ph.D., F.R.C.P., F.R.S.C., F.I. Biol., Prof of Nutrition at London University

What's so bad about sugar?

Refined sugar[21] significantly lowers vibrations in animals and humans, and can weaken physical defenses in numerous ways, leading to dis-ease. In his book on the Ninxia Wolfberry, Discovery of the Ultimate Super Food, Dr. Gary Young writes:

"One of the most important predictors of life expectancy is the blood sugar level. The higher and longer sugar levels stay, the more cellular damage accrues. The culprit is known as a Maillard reaction, where sugar forms irreversible chemical bonds with proteins, and renders them useless and inert inside the body. As more and more proteins become complexed with sugars (sugar coated), the more dead tissues increase."

The Maillard reaction is a non-enzymatic browning that occurs when heat, amino acid and sugar interact. The sugar of fruit in its natural state will not have the same harmful effect, because it is more complex and more complete. The complex chains of glycemic (sugar) molecules coupled with the fiber of fruit take longer to be digested and filtered into the bloodstream, and therefore will not "spike" it with glucose the way

---

[21] See "Sugar Blues" by William Dufty, "Get the Sugar Out" by Louise Gittleman. And "Lick the Sugar Habit" by Dr. Nancy Appleton

processed sugar will—given the person eating the fruit is not diabetic or otherwise low in insulin.

In the above quote from Dr Young we see one scenario that causes the heart, liver, kidneys, and pancreas to have to work extra hard to bring the body back to homeostasis. In this situation, one cannot expect to resonate on higher vibrational planes, and that's just the proverbial tip of the sugar iceberg.

Refined sugar actually feeds cancer

There are several factors associated with the proliferation of cancer cells; processed sugar is one of them. In 1931 Nobel laureate Dr. Otto Warburg, PhD demonstrated that cancer cells show an increase in **anaerobic glycolysis**. Anaerobic = living without oxygen; glycolysis = the metabolic breakdown of sugar for energy.

Our bodies are perfectly capable of handling normal glucose metabolism. But instead of processing glucose the way healthy cells do, cancer cells in anaerobic glycolysis, cause the glucose to ferment. This fermented sugar eliminates oxygen in the cells. Copious amounts of lactic acid as a by-product of fermenting sugar are available fuel for the cancer cells. Healthy cells require oxygen for glycolysis; malignant cells thrive in its absence. Sugar (glucose) is very acid forming when it is metabolized; it is pure carbohydrate (Carbon, Oxygen and Hydrogen) with no vitamins, proteins or minerals to assist in metabolism.

In 1957, Dr William Coda Martin labeled refined sugar as the "sweetest poison of all". In one of his articles he states:

"The body cannot utilize this refined starch and carbohydrate unless the depleted proteins, vitamins and minerals are present. Nature supplies these elements in each plant in quantities sufficient to metabolize the carbohydrate in that particular plant. There is no excess for other added carbohydrates.

Incomplete carbohydrate metabolism results in the formation of 'toxic metabolite' such as pyruvic acid and abnormal sugars containing five carbon atoms. Pyruvic acid accumulates in the brain and nervous system and the abnormal sugars in the red blood cells. These toxic metabolites interfere with the respiration of the cells. They cannot get sufficient oxygen to survive and function normally. In time, some of the cells die. This interferes with the function of a part of the body and is the beginning of degenerative disease.

... Excessive sugar has a strong mal-effect on the functioning of the brain. The key to orderly brain

function is glutamic acid, a vital compound found in many vegetables."[22]

"The B vitamins play a major role in dividing glutamic acid into antagonistic-complementary compounds which produce a "proceed" or "control" response in the brain. B vitamins are also manufactured by symbiotic bacteria, which live in our intestines. When refined sugar is taken daily, these bacteria wither and die, and our stock of B vitamins gets very low. Too much sugar makes one sleepy; our ability to calculate and remember is lost."[23]

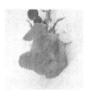

---

[22]From "Dangers of Refined Sugar", Global Health Center
[23]See internet article "Refined Sugar, the Sweetest Poison of All" by William Martin.

Stolen sweets are always sweeter;
Stolen kisses much completer;
Stolen looks are nice in chapels;
Stolen, stolen be your apples.

- James Leigh Hunt, [Fairies' Song, 1830)

Sugar intake causes a flood of insulin and other stress hormones into the bloodstream, which in turn tax the heart, pancreas, kidneys and liver. The level of vibration frequencies, the potency of life-force and the overall condition of these vital organs weigh heavily on our ability live and to express health and wellness. Extended high amounts of sugar in the bloodstream not only tax these organs, but will eventually cause them to enlarge from the stress of being overworked, which is a precursor to several life-threatening conditions.

Understanding the importance of steering away from refined cane sugar, some concerned parents turn to honey and/or isolated fructose (sold in health food stores) as alternatives for their children. This may not be the best thing to do, because being bereft of minerals, vitamins or enzymes, pure isolated fructose—like sugar, delivers high amounts of empty calories to the body. In addition, continuous use of fructose can cause liver damage, because unlike glucose, which is metabolized in every cell in the body, fructose is metabolized only in the liver.

Children younger than one year old should not have honey at all; honey has microscopic botulism spores that could be a serious threat to their very young body systems. In addition, much of today's honey is depleted of many nutrients, because the honey bees are no longer resting during the winter without food, which is what would normally happen in nature. Instead, they are fed refined sugar to cause them to continuously produce more honey for the industry.

On the other hand, the natural, complete sugar in raw fruit will not cause a negative reaction, but will actually help support the body's healing processes; this form of sugar is what the body can thrive on.

Dr. Nancy Appleton, PhD, is the author of the book *Lick the Sugar Habit*. She compiled the following list entitled *"78 ways Sugar can Ruin Your Health"* from several medical journals and other scientific publications:[24]

1. Sugar can suppress the immune system.
2. Sugar can upset the body's mineral balance.
3. Sugar can cause hyperactivity, anxiety, concentration difficulties, and crankiness in children.
4. Sugar can cause drowsiness and decreased activity in children.
5. Sugar can adversely affect children's school grades.

---

[24] www.nancyappleton.com

6. Sugar can produce a significant rise in triglycerides.
7. Sugar contributes to a weakened defense against bacterial infection.
8. Sugar can cause kidney damage.
9. Sugar can reduce helpful high density cholesterol (HDLs).
10. Sugar can promote an elevation of harmful cholesterol (LDLs).
11. Sugar may lead to chromium deficiency.
12. Sugar can cause copper deficiency.
13. Sugar interferes with absorption of calcium and magnesium.
14. Sugar may lead to cancer of the breast, ovaries, prostate, and rectum.
15. Sugar can cause colon cancer, with an increased risk in women.
16. Sugar can be a risk factor in gall bladder cancer.
17. Sugar can increase fasting levels of blood glucose.
18. Sugar can weaken eyesight.
19. Sugar raises the level of a neurotransmitter called serotonin, which can narrow blood vessels.
20. Sugar can cause hypoglycemia.
21. Sugar can produce an acidic stomach.
22. Sugar can raise adrenaline levels in children.
23. Sugar can increase the risk of coronary heart disease.
24. Sugar can speed the aging process, causing wrinkles and grey hair.

25. Sugar can lead to alcoholism.

26. Sugar can promote tooth decay.

27. Sugar can contribute to weight gain and obesity.

28. High intake of sugar increases the risk of Crohn's disease and ulcerative colitis.

29. Sugar can cause a raw, inflamed intestinal tract in persons with gastric or duodenal ulcers.

30. Sugar can cause arthritis

31. Sugar can cause asthma.

32. Sugar can cause candidiasis (yeast infection).

33. Sugar can lead to the formation of gallstones.

34. Sugar can lead to the formation of kidney stones.

35. Sugar can cause ischemic heart disease.

36. Sugar can cause appendicitis.

37. Sugar can exacerbate the symptoms of multiple sclerosis.

38. Sugar can indirectly cause hemorrhoids.

39. Sugar can cause varicose veins.

40. Sugar can elevate glucose and insulin responses in oral contraception users.

41. Sugar can lead to periodontal disease.

42. Sugar can contribute to osteoporosis.

43. Sugar contributes to saliva acidity.

44. Sugar can cause a decrease in insulin sensitivity.

45. Sugar leads to decreased glucose tolerance.

46. Sugar can decrease growth hormone.

47. Sugar can increase total cholesterol.

48. Sugar can increase systolic blood pressure.

49. Sugar can change the structure of protein causing interference with protein absorption.
50. Sugar causes food allergies.
51. Sugar can contribute to diabetes.
52. Sugar can cause toxemia during pregnancy.
53. Sugar can contribute to eczema in children.
54. Sugar can cause cardiovascular disease.
55. Sugar can impair the structure of DNA.
56. Sugar can cause cataracts.
57. Sugar can cause emphysema.
58. Sugar can cause atherosclerosis.
59. Sugar can cause free radical formation in the bloodstream.
60. Sugar lowers the enzymes' ability to function.
61. Sugar can cause loss of tissue elasticity and function.
62. Sugar can cause liver cells to divide, increasing the size of the liver.
63. Sugar can increase the amount of fat in the liver.
64. Sugar can increase kidney size and produce pathological changes in the kidney.
65. Sugar can overstress the pancreas, causing damage.
66. Sugar can increase the body's fluid retention.
67. Sugar can cause constipation.
68. Sugar can cause myopia (nearsightedness).
69. Sugar can compromise the lining of the capillaries.
70. Sugar can cause hypertension.

71. Sugar can cause headaches, including migraines.
72. Sugar can cause an increase in delta, alpha and theta brain waves, which can alter the mind's ability to think clearly.
73. Sugar can cause depression.
74. Sugar can increase insulin responses in those consuming high-sugar diets compared to low sugar diets.
75. Sugar increases bacterial fermentation in the colon.
76. Sugar can cause hormonal imbalance.
77. Sugar can increase blood platelet adhesiveness which increases risk of blood clots.
78. Sugar increases the risk of Alzheimer Disease.

"I pity them greatly, but I must be mum, for how could we do without sugar and rum?"

"Pity for Poor Africans,"
- William Cowper, 1788

Again, **Organic,** raw food (also known as "live food") has a much higher vibration frequency than cooked food. One reason is because the electrolytes (sodium, chloride, potassium, calcium, magnesium) in raw food are still intact. All fruits and vegetables have the delicate enzymes that we discussed earlier. They are vital defense system regulators that your body uses to create vitamins and minerals. A temperature above 116-118 degrees Fahrenheit destroys many of those enzymes.

According to Dr Edward Howell, renowned enzyme specialist for more than 50 years:

"Enzymes have vital life force that initiates biochemical interactions."

In other words, enzyme activity is not only life sustaining activity; it is actually life *creating* activity. Without enzymes there is no life. You can insure that you get a sufficient amount of enzymes by having plenty of raw organic fruit, vegetables and their fresh juices.

Remember, you are renewing yourself daily.
As your vibrations attain higher levels, your hair, skin, nails and entire countenance will resonate with and reflect a noticeably healthier cellular structure fostered by the enzymes of live foods.

"To laugh often and much, to win the respect of intelligent people, and the affection of children… to leave the world a better place… To know even one life has breathed easier because you have lived – that is to have succeeded"

- Ralph Waldo Emerson (1803-1882)

Breathing

Breathing is the most important thing you do to nourish your cells, and keep you in this present consciousness envelope; it is your fundamental connection to the physical realm. You can live several days without food, but only a few minutes without air. We inhale about 15 times per minute, using only 12 percent of our lung capacity.

Most of us don't realize that we actually process minerals e.g. potassium calcium, magnesium, etc. directly *from the air we breathe*. Breathing exercises can increase your lung capacity, activate your lymphatic vessels, lower your blood pressure, and substantially raise your level of vibrations; Breathing is the way we receive and give, share and participate with and in the Universe. When you inhale, you take in solaric gases primarily nitrogen (about 78%), oxygen (21%), and including argon, helium, carbon dioxide, and other gases. The air is filtered, warmed and moistened as it enters into the passages of your nostrils. The majority of these gases are carried into your lungs, your blood and the rest of your body, where the transformation of chemical compounds takes place—where the actual *breathing* takes place. When you exhale, waste in the form of carbon dioxide is carried out of your body.

Your Breath is Focused Energy

By incorporating a Yogic exercise of conscious breathing, you can create internal chemical changes to increase your mental awareness, facilitate healing, eliminate emotional blocks, soothe your spirit and give you access to renewed creativity. All of this is possible because your breath is focused energy, and the more you focus upon it, the more effective it becomes:

Through conscious breathing we also

- Eliminate seventy percent of our toxic bodily waste
- Burn fat and lose weight
- Reduce blood acid levels
- Improve our complexion
- Reduce water retention
- Release endorphins into the blood

Breathing is an excellent way to manage that all – too-familiar daily stress we experience.

We breathe with the entire body, not just with the lungs. Earlier, I briefly alluded to the fact that the food we eat is not our only source of nutrients. In reality, we are not composed of the food we eat, but of the gases that our bodies convert the food into. This is the main reason we are able to live for days, weeks—even months without eating, but only a few minutes at the most without air.

(Believe it not, there *are* actually a few living Breatharians on earth today.)

Breathing is naturally, a major component of the healing process; but, as practicing Yogis know, with *conscious, purposeful* breathing we can generate higher vibration nerve-currents. By regulating the breath, we can also learn to regulate the effectiveness of our brain, as well as our other inner organs. (I often refer to the "Hippies" of the 60's and 70's, who, being high on marijuana, would say, "Raaaaiiiisse your vibrraations, maaaaan!" They had the right idea—too bad they just didn't realize they were systematically lowering their own cerebral vibrations at that very moment.)

Unfortunately, there are many varying things that cause us to breathe shallowly, and to even (unwittingly) hold our breath. Anxiety, fear, anger, grief, negative emotions et al, are major culprits, along with poor posture, and lack of exercise. Once again, breathing exercises will remedy the resulting low levels of oxygen, and restore vibrancy to the internal organs.

"The only thing better than singing, is more singing."

- Ella Fitzgerald, (1917-1996)

Singing is yet another way to increase your oxygen intake, and raise your emotional vibration-frequency. You may also find that singing will cause you to align with several of the 7 Steps at one time.

While singing a favorite song, you immediately bring your inner, more subtle vibrations up to meet with the higher frequencies of that which you create with your voice; you release negative emotions; you also synchronize your pineal and throat chakras with your heart chakra, allowing them to resonate with and participate in even more positive vibrations. The throat chakra holds the regulating frequencies for healthy thyroid and adrenal function, which will positively affect your entire being.

Physically, just the mechanics of singing alone will force you to breathe more deeply, and to receive the benefits of increased blood-levels of oxygen.

Note: All of the above mentioned Essential Oils are oxygen carriers.

Exercise

Important: As you practice, do not tighten any part of your body. Remain totally relaxed.

1. When you first become conscious in the morning, before getting up, take 3 slow, deep, but *very gentle* breaths, making sure to exhale fully.

2. Sit on the side of the bed, with your shoulders relaxed, and back straight, but not stiff. With your lips closed, your tongue gently touching the roof of your mouth, with one finger, close one nostril, and take a deep breath in through the other nostril. Hold for a second or two; exhale through the nostril that was held. Inhale through the nostril that you just exhaled out of. Repeat 2 more times, alternating nostrils.

3. Inhale fully through the nose, while lifting your shoulders up to your ears. As you drop your shoulders, exhale with your mouth open, making the aspirated sound "huh", without using your voice—only air, no sound should come out.
    Repeat 2 more times

7 Steps to Healing & Wellness

At night, before lying down, reverse the order of the exercises, ending with 3 slow gentle breaths. Then lie on your back; be completely still; bring your awareness to every aspect of your being, beginning with your feet, ankles, knees, etc., all the way to the top of your head, while noticing and releasing any tension therein.

As you feel yourself relaxing more and more, bring your attention to your abdomen, and notice how it rises and falls with each breath. Try not to "make" it move, just notice the movement.

Breathe; relax; empty; enjoy the breath; release the tension, and have a good night's sleep.

"Music is the truest form of art... Therefore true poets, they who are seers seek to express the universe in terms of music...the singer has everything within him. The notes come out from his very life; they are not materials gathered from outside"

Rabindranath Taqor, (1861-1941)

To experience pain is inevitable

To suffer is optional

Most of us sing only when we are already in a good mood. When we're not, we tend to want to hold on to whatever source of irritation we've encountered. We would rather wallow in the loop of painful thought remembrances than choose the freedom of forgiveness. This is a powerful and potentially debilitating force of habit. To resonate with vitality in your wellness zone, you can raise your vibrations with a song and replace that habit.

When you are happy and/or content, you will broadcast and resonate with happiness and contentment. This doesn't mean that you will (or even should) always wear a smile on your face; it's just helpful for you to be more conscious as to what you are resonating with at any given moment. Again, it is a choice that you make.

"Trying creates impossibilities, letting go creates what is desired."

\- Stalking Wolf, Apache elder

Essential oils are co-resonant vibrational supporters with the harmonic energies of the earth and the Great Pyramids of Giza

Essential Oil Recommendations

I cannot over-emphasize the importance of using therapeutic grade essential oils as opposed to so-called "pure", "organic", "natural" or any other grade oils. I do not use nor do I recommend them. With other oils, you cannot expect the same results; and you may even get negative reactions. Throughout the book, wherever essential oils are mentioned, I am referring to therapeutic grade essential oils exclusively.

The chemical constituents of therapeutic grade Essential Oils are extensive and considerably diverse. Because there are so many of them, you will be able to find an Essential Oil to help with virtually every health issue you may encounter.

Therapeutic grade essential oils are anti-fungal, antibacterial, antiseptic, anti-inflammatory, antimicrobial, antiparasitic, anti-depressant, antiviral and analgesic.

For an in depth catalog of applications for each of the categories named above, see *The Essential Oil*

Desk or Pocket Reference by Essential Science Publishing[25].

There are many high vibrational essential oils that directly affect the emotional resonance field—not only of humans, but of animals as well. A few of them are: Frankincense, Neroli, Orange, Tangerine, Melissa and Ylang-Ylang.

Please note: Although these essential oils are GRAS (Generally Regarded As Safe) by the Food and Drug Administration (FDA), and can be taken internally as dietary supplements, they should not be used without the supervision of a health care practitioner who knows the proper indications and contra-indications for the use of such EO's. In the case of pregnancy, check with your Aromatherapist before using.

One of the many ways that Essential Oils are used to affect the body is by diffusing them into the air for inhalation. By simply inhaling an Essential Oil we can positively affect our health, because the molecules of the oil travel directly into the brain, lungs and bloodstream via the olfactory nerves. When essential oils are placed on the skin—especially on the soles of the feet—

[25]www.essentialscience.net To order essential oils, go to www.healbytouch.com.

they can be in the blood-stream within 3-6 seconds.

Capillaries (microscopic blood vessels) maintain a protective barrier that will only allow certain substances from our bloodstream through to our brain and spinal fluid. This is called the "blood-brain barrier". The blood-brain barrier is extremely selective in what it will allow through; it's so selective in fact, that it does not allow medication through that scientists believe would "cure" degenerative dis-eases of the brain.

Some Essential Oils contain valuable substances called sesquiterpones and sesquiterpines.
They have the ability to cross the blood-brain barrier with their ionized, oxygenating molecules. This also has significance, as it makes it possible to positively affect brain function through the use of these Essential Oils.

Most of the data below is extracted from the *Essential Oils Desk Reference*, with a few minor additions from my own personal research and experience with EO's...

Frankincense – Boswella (B)
Frankincense is an oleo-gum-resin extracted from the Boswella (B) trees of East Africa. The different strains of Frankincense - (B. Carteri, B Sacra, B Papyrifera, B. Frereana; and from India

(B Serrata) will offer slight variations in the aromatic profile of the oil.

Frankincense contains sesquiterpines. It permeates the blood-brain barrier and stimulates the limbic system, hypothalamus, pineal and pituitary glands.

It is...

- a DNA repairer
- a promoter of spiritual awareness
- mentioned in the Ebers Papyrus, an ancient medical record of Kemet.
- an anti-tumoral
- a natural anti-oxidant
- an anti-depressant
- a bactericide
- an anti-inflammatory and
- a muscle relaxant
- an anti-asthmatic

Used for...

- cuts, sores, insect bites
- cancer
- depression
- colds, flu, respiratory infections
- stiff, sore muscles
- as an astringent

- heavy menstruation

Fragrant influence on olfactory nerves

- Increases spiritual awareness
- Promotes meditation
- Uplifts spirits
- Improves attitudes

Neroli absolute – (Citrus aurantium)

– Extracted from blossoms of the Orange trees of North East Africa – mainly of Morocco and Tunisia.

It is (an)...

- Anti-parasitic
- Anti-depressant
- cytophylactic

- Hypotensive (lowers blood pressure)
- Digestive tonic
- Historically used by Kemetians to as a spiritual uplifter. Today it is also used to encourage skin cell regeneration

Used for...

- frigidity
- shock

- hysteria
- insomnia
- anxiety
- as a skin conditioner (scars, stretch marks, thread veins, wrinkles)

Fragrant influence on olfactory nerves:

"A natural relaxant used to treat depression and anxiety. It strengthens and stabilizes the emotions, and uplifts and inspires the hopeless, encouraging confidence, courage, joy, peace and sensuality. It brings everything into focus at the moment."[26]

Note: All citrus oils are photosynthesizing – meaning they create carbohydrates from carbon dioxide and hydrogen (precipitating water), using solar energy.

This could cause the skin to burn. For this reason, it is advisable to avoid using citrus oils several hours before exposing the skin to direct sunlight. Some experts recommend 72 hours, others say 12hrs, or only at night. (Personally, I've never experienced this effect when using these oils and going directly into sunlight, but I must caution you nevertheless).

---

[26]Pg 70, Essential Oil Desk Reference, Essential Science Publishing

Orange (Citrus sinensis)

Plant origin – USA, South Africa, Italy, China

Cold pressed from the rind

It is (a, an)...

- anti-tumoral
- antiseptic
- antibacterial
- relaxant
- anti-coagulant-
- anti-spasmodic
- circulatory stimulant
- rich in limonene, which has been extensively studied for its ability to combat tumor growth in over 50 clinical studies
- to encourage a peaceful state of mind
- as a supplement, boosts the defense system

Fragrant influence:

Uplifting anti-depressant

Used for...

Arteriosclerosis
- hypertension
- cancer
- insomnia
- collagen formation
- fluid retention
- an air purifier
- indoor insect repellent
- a hospital and household cleanser

Tangerine (Citrus Nobilis, C. Reticulata, C. Madurensis, C. Unshiu, C. Deliciosa)

Plant origin: Originally China, USA, South Africa

Cold pressed from the rind

It is (a, an)...

- anti-tumoral
- relaxant
- anti-spasmodic
- digestive aid
- circulatory enhancer
- rich in limonene
- cytophylactic

Used for...

- anxiety
- obesity
- liver problems
- fluid retention
- digestive problems
- parasites
- diarrhea, constipation

Fragrant influence on olfactory nerves

- promotes happiness
- calming
- soothes nervousness
- reduces depression
- boosts bodily defenses

Melissa - Melissa officinalis
Also known as Lemon, Sweet, Common and Bee Balm

Plant origin – Utah, Idaho, France, Mediterranean region

Steam distilled from leaves and flowers

Properties:

- anti-inflammatory
- anti-viral
- relaxant
- hypotensive
- anti-depressant
- antispasmodic
- diaphoretic
- febrifuge (anti-pyretic)
- carminative

Used for...

- herpes simplex
- depression
- insomnia
- dyspepsia
- anxiety, panic
- headaches
- painful menstrual cycles

Fragrant influence on olfactory nerves

- Brings out gentle characteristics in people
- calming
- uplifting
- balances emotions

Ylang Ylang – Cananga odorata

Steam distilled from flowers
Plant Origin
Commodores, Indonesia, Philippines
Ylang Ylang means "Flower of Flowers". It is traditionally strewn on the beds of newlywed couples.

Properties:

Contains sesquiterpines
- antispasmodic
- vasodilating
- anti-diabetic
- anti-inflammatory
- anti-parasitic
- anti-parasitic
- antiseptic
- hypotensive
- nervine

Used for...
- Cardiac arrhythmia
- anxiety
- depression
- hypertension
- hair loss
- intestinal problems

- frigidity, impotence
- low self esteem

Fragrant influence on olfactory nerves

- Balances male – female energies
- enhances spiritual attunement
- combats anger
- encourages mental focus
- filters out negative energy
- restores confidence and peace

Clinical studies are constantly being conducted to reveal the efficacy of essential oils for different pathologies. Many of those studies focus on their effects on depression—a major condition of consistently low vibrations.

Studies at the University of Vienna have shown through functional imaging that cineol—one of the primary constituents in some of the oils—stimulates blood flow and activity in the limbic (emotional) region of the brain; another series of studies conducted at the Department of Psychiatry at the Mie University of Medicine in Japan revealed that inhaling the essential oil of lemon reduced depression *and* stress.

The few essential oils that we listed above have the ability to do exactly that, as they assist the body in raising internal Resonance frequencies. They have been used for many millennia—from the ancient Kemetians to today—to help us resonate more completely with our higher inner consciousness

"Having soon discovered to be great, I must appear so, and therefore studiously avoided mixing in society, and wrapped myself in mystery, devoting my time to fasting and prayer."

- Nat Turner

Fasting to Raise Your Vibrations

Caution:
If you are underweight (by 10 pounds or more), pregnant, or diagnosed with a serious illness, you should not fast without the guidance of a health care practitioner. Everyone should consult with a doctor or health care practitioner before attempting a multiple-day fast.

The term "fast" has many definitions. As an adjective, it can mean firm, swift, sudden, prompt, hasty, etc. As a verb, it means to stop, or cease from an activity – especially from eating.

There are numerous benefits to fasting; some are immediately recognized; others are not so obvious. We age when more cells die than new ones are being built. When we fast, the reverse occurs; the rate of cellular regeneration increases, and digestive metabolic energy is re-routed to wherever we need it the most for healing.

Fasting will raise your spiritual and bioelectric vibrations, facilitate healing, lead you away from a mundane existence, and help you to resonate with your higher self. When we fast we lose excess weight, cleanse the blood, detoxify the body, create healthier cells and body tissue, and support the heart, pancreas, liver, gallbladder and kidneys.

Again, if you have health issues, or if you intend to fast for several days, consult a specialist for guidance.

"The best of all medicines
is Fasting"

- Benjamin Franklin

According to fasting expert Paavo Airola, we can fast as long as 40 days on water, and up to 100 days on juices. To go farther would be putting ourselves in danger. Again, multiple-day fasting should be done with the guidance of a health care practitioner.

After 2 or 3 days of fasting we begin to experience **autolysis**. Autolysis is the process of digesting our own cells, for energy. (We don't really "burn" cells)

The Divine Intelligence that guides and operates the life force within knows which cells we need least. When fasting, we first digest damaged, mutated (potentially cancerous), dead and aged cells; then we convert carbohydrates, fat, and protein into usable glucose. As we get rid of dead cells and other waste, the residual nutrients in our blood can more readily nourish our healthy cells; we begin producing new cells at a faster pace, and those cells are less likely to become damaged. That's why we tend to look younger. In this process, we actually *are* younger; our senses are sharper, and we have more energy because we have conserved digestive enzymes, and we are internally renewed.

Fasting allows the body to cleanses away internal debris

To cease speaking for a specified number of days is considered a form of fasting by some; it's a fast from vocal participation, which to some extent can be a trying experience.

The ancient wise ones of many cultures taught their students and Initiates the value of being completely silent for extended periods of time. They wanted their students to perfect the ability to hear their own inner voice, and observe the chaotic world around them without feeling the need to participate in the chaos.

Vocal fasting assists in the rest and recuperation process; it can also guide you into a uniquely meditative state. Like the students, initiates and Monks mentioned above, through silence you too can extricate yourself from participating in the noise and chaos of a cacophonous world. It can help you hear *your* inner voice, while you observe yourself and the world around you. Practicing silence is another form of practicing yoga[27].

We all can benefit from practicing silence. Teachers and children in school would have less stress and accomplish more if they were allowed 15 to 30 minutes a day of peaceful silence.

---

[27] Yoga means "union". Practicing yoga can strengthen you physically and spiritually.

Have you ever wondered why your "health-nut" friends fast so often? Maybe they know that 75 to 80% of our daily energy is used to digest large meals. When we fast, our energy turns from the heavy task of digestion to purification, healing and spiritual rejuvenation, thus we are freer to resonate more consistently with the higher self.

In order for the spiritual aspect of a fast to be effective, we must consciously cease from participating in the lower vibrational realms of thought. Ideally, we isolate ourselves from the world outside, and go deeper within to commune with and learn from the Divine Self, or the "One Most High".

We may not always be able to physically remove ourselves from our environment, but we *can* do so mentally. If you've never meditated before, a minimum of 5 minutes of meditation each day is a good way to begin, and then increase the time as you become accustomed to the practice.

"When the stomach is full it is easy to talk of fasting"

St Jerome

"The philosopher is like a man fasting in the midst of universal intoxication. He alone perceives the illusion of which all creatures are the willing playthings; he is less duped than his neighbor by his own nature. He judges more sanely, he sees things as they are. It is in this that his liberty consists — in the ability to see clearly and soberly, in the power of mental record".

Henri Frederic Amiel
1821 - 1881

Acknowledge your inner light

You are a being of light. Before you dismiss this as only an esoteric statement, you should know that scientists (have) proved this fact. Biophysicist Fritz-Albert Popp discovered that we emit a permanent current of light photons. Other Russian scientists have found light photons in human Cranial Sacral fluid[28] (CSF, also called CranioSacral Fluid). In his book *Craniosacral Biodynamics* Franklyn Sills thoroughly explains the constitutional qualities of CSF. Speaking of the fluid matrix within the body he states:

"...The fluids have been seen to convey bioelectric or bio-magnetic information throughout the body at lightning speeds..."

Everything that we see, touch, feel and recognize has its genesis in the metaphysical realm. Your body is a product of metaphysical processes composed of interlacing light frequencies, crystallizing by degrees into the elemental properties of organic matter. You are a being of crystal light; your blood is liquid crystal; it is a flowing river of light, directly connected to the light of Cosmic Intelligence. From this river, the

---

[28] Cranial Sacral fluid is the fluid that surrounds your brain and spinal cord.

subtle fluid wavelengths of light that nurture and sustain the body and mind resonate to feed and instruct the cellular networks on different levels of vibration. These wavelengths of light are comprised of light photons; light photons are messengers, transporting vital instructions to every cell in the body.

So now we see that light photons are in your blood *and* in your CranioSacral Fluid (CSF), and they both communicate directly with every cell in your collective body—your mind-body-spirit matrix.

The detectable light photons permeating our CranialSacral Fluid for example, are constituents of this flowing river of Cosmic Light, and are sustained by higher, faster and lighter vibrations than those that are found in other parts of the body.

Regular fasting and meditation (be it once a season, once a week or once a month) enhance the resonance quotient of the light-body matrix in conjunction with the various aspects of the physical body. By raising its vibrational frequency, they also provide a substantial connection to one's innermost being. This can be detected in and by the quality of the flow of the CranialSacral Fluid.

CranioSacral Health practitioners connect and communicate with the innermost core of the individual via the ebb and flow of CSF when we do CranioSacral Biodynamic work. Franklyn Sills calls that innermost core Primary Respiration, or "The Breath of Life." We can detect and observe any obstructions to that flow, and through a higher vibrational energetic connection, participate in the re-establishing of vibrant health.

It is a most rewarding experience to be a privileged bystander as healing occurs.

*Your inner light
is a mode of communication*

You are a magnificent
Electromagnetic Conductor

Mobile Telephones

Cellular mobile telephones (cell phones) emit what is called low-density, pulsed, microwave radiation (MWR). It is the same radiation as is used in the microwave oven. Microwave ovens cook food by passing an electromagnetic wave through it; the heat is produced with the absorption of microwave energy by the water molecules in the food. Since we know that we are electromagnetic conductors, that brain activity is electromagnetic activity, and that over 75% of our bodies consist of water, we should understand the obvious implications of MWR as it inter-acts with human brain cells.

From the Telephone

In addition to the microwaves from the handset of the phone, currents of electricity emanate from the battery. These currents of erratic, chaotic electric waves can (and do) interfere with the electrical processes of the brain.

Physicist Dr. Gerald Hyland wrote an article on this subject in the British Medical Journal *The Lancet.* In it he explains:

"A handset that is in operation also has a low-frequency magnetic field (EMF) associated, not with

the emitted microwaves, but with surges of electric current from the battery that are necessary to implement "time division multiple access "(TDMA)".

Electromagnetic Interference is an undeniable reality that we must contend with. Cordless and cellular phones represent only one aspect of that interference[29]. To resonate in the best of health, we must be circumspect in the use of all electrical appliances. It is also advisable to:

• Get an RF3 protective headset.
• Restrict your use of ALL phones to calls that are really necessary.
• Unplug and cover the outlets in your bedroom at night particularly when your vibrations are low, and when you're not feeling well. (The Pineal gland is more susceptible to those harmful rays when we are asleep).
• Sleep with your head facing North (think of a compass that aligns with the magnetic field of the earth).
• Limit the use of a micro-wave oven for food preparation.(You may consider eliminating it altogether, knowing how it also totally destroys live enzyme activity)
• Wash your hands after using computers and other electrical appliances.

---

[29]Please read "The Body Electric" by Robert Becker, and "Electromagnetic Pollution" by Dr Sabina M Devita. Visit

Equilibrium is what
you truly seek

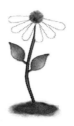

Chapter 6
The Fourth Step
Equilibrium

The Principle of Polarity

"This principle embodies the truth that 'everything is dual'; 'everything has two poles; everything has its pair of opposites',"

The Kybalion, p32

WITHOUT OPPOSING ASPECTS OF A GIVEN entity, it would not exist. There would be no inside without an outside, no hot without cold, no top without a bottom, or physical without the spiritual.

Polarity is the Kemetic/Hermetic law that generates and sustains equilibrium. Your inner biological mechanisms are constantly seeking balance, in both **dynamic** and **static** forms. Dynamic equilibrium is the balance between opposite chemical reactions, and static equilibrium—the simple ability to stand without falling.

Maat is one of several Kemetic words that can be used to depict equilibrium. (Actually, some of the other words can be more literally translated as "balance", but Maat has become the more popular word, due to the way it is depicted). In Mdu Ntr (pronounced "Medu Netcher), the original language of Kemet, the root word "maa" literally means "true" or "truth". It also means, "to see". Maat can also be translated "that which is straight". It is sometimes depicted on the walls of Kemet as a woman with a feather on her head, outstretched arms with wings, or holding the scales of balance in one of her hands.

Maat is a detached principle of equilibrium and law, not a (an) judgment, emotion or feeling. It is the law of measures whereby the mind of the Universe seeks its central point of reference within all things.

Other English words that can be translated as Maat are balance, righteousness, rightness and reciprocity. Metaphysically, their definitions are very much the same; they all represent the equalizing of energies and the answering of the essence of unspoken questions.

"Be careful of what you ask for" the axiom goes. This is sound advice, because you could be consciously or unconsciously seeking Maat (to "see") or balance in what you request of the Universe, and may not be prepared for the reality of the mental, physical or emotional metamorphosis required as a prerequisite to the requested end result. Maat will bring clarity and balance, pain or pleasure notwithstanding.

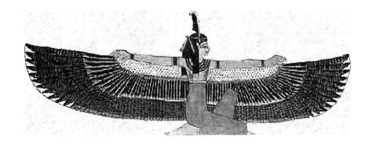

Maat

"Endj hr K Maat"

"I seek your counsel Maat"

"The breaking wave and the muscle as it contracts obey the same law. Delicate line gathers the body's strength in a bold balance. Shall my soul meet so severe a curve journeying on its way to form?"

- Dag Hammarskjöld
1905 - 1961

Equilibrium/Maat

Deep within your tissues, you have receptors that monitor and report any physical changes that may occur in the body for the sole purpose of maintaining internal and proprioceptive[30] equilibrium.

Your inner ear contains several parts that together are called your vestibular apparatus, or system. It has fluid canals that send signals to your brain. At the same time, in the process of proprioception, your muscles are sending signals to your brain via your nervous system. In response, your brain informs your muscles of the need to contract or relax where needed. Proprioception is the subjective consciousness that operates to allow you (for example) to touch your nose with your eyes closed.

When you bend forward the muscles in the front of your body (your "flexors") contract, while those in the back (your extensors) relax and stretch. Even when you are standing or sitting still, your brain, nerves and muscles are working to prevent you from falling over. It's all in the process of maintaining physical equilibrium.

---

[30]Proprioception: The ability to sense the position, location and orientation of all parts of the body.

Metaphysically your intent, thoughts and agreements set the template that enables you to maintain psycho-spiritual and emotional equilibrium.

"So divinely is the world organized that every one of us, in our place and time, is in balance with everything else."

Johann Wolfgang von Goethe
- 1749 - 1832

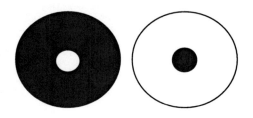

Yin Yang

Maat as Yin Yang
Cold/hot, soft/hard, round/pointed;
dull/sharp, empty/full, blue/red,
slow/fast, thin/thick, long/short...

We can observe all of the above polarities being expressed at different times and in varying degrees by the human body, as it pursues equilibrium.

The very foundation of all Natural and Wholistic disciplines of ancient peoples – Ayurveda, Native Healing, Shiatsu, Qigong, Tui Na, Yoga, Tai Chi, TCM, etc – is **balance.** Many today are learning and practicing the basic principles of Traditional Chinese Medicine (TCM). Thousands of years ago, these principles emerged from Kemet in the fundamental teachings of Maat.

One of the major theories of TCM is called the *5 Element Theory.* In it, each of the visceral organs of the body is aligned with either the element of wood, fire, earth, metal or water; they also correspond with 5 emotional temperaments, and the 4 seasons, which resonate with specific colors. Regarding the 5 Element theory, author Giovanni Maciocia writes:

"...Some of the earliest references to the elements do not call them "elements" at all but either "seats of government" (Fu) or "ability, talent, material" (cai)..."[31]

It can also be said that a given element governs a particular organ. Every emotion as well, has a

---

[31] The Foundations of Chinese Medicine – Maciocia, p16.

corresponding organ that it affects more directly than the rest of the body.

TCM is a philosophy rich in ancient wisdom and good old (not-so) common sense; to get a solid inner, under and overstanding of its use in maintaining optimal health, we would need about 500 more pages, the opportunity to sit with a Chinese Master for 5 years, and at least 20 years of practice. For our purposes of exploring aspects of Equilibrium, I simply make mention of the very basic rudiments of TCM.

"There is vitality, a life-force, energy, a quickening that is translated through you into action, and because there is only one of you in all of time this expression is unique. And if you block it, it will never exist through any other medium and be lost. The world will not have it! It is not your business to determine how good it is nor how it compares with other expressions. It is your business to keep it yours clearly and directly, to keep the channel open."

- Martha Graham

There are several names for the energetic life force that invisibly flows from the single innermost point of light throughout all aspects of your being. It can be detected in your astral, ethereal and somatic "bodies". In India it is called "kundalini"; the ancient Kemites called it "kha"; the Japanese say "ki" (pronounced kee) and the Chinese say "qi", (pronounced "chee"). Whatever the nomenclature, this energetic life force moves along specific channels called "meridians". It flows in and out of your organs, and gathers together at specific points of vortex-references called "chakras", to use the popular Sanskrit word for "wheel".

Many things influence Qi; among them are food, sleep, colors, electricity, thoughts and emotions. We use an enormous amount of energy when we sustain extreme emotional moods. Too much joy (yes there is such a state of being) can throw you out of balance, and affect the flow of your heart-qi.

Fire – Heart, Spleen, Small Intestine
Earth – Stomach, Pancreas
Metal – Lung, Large Intestine
Water – Kidney, Bladder
Wood – Liver, Gallbladder

Having an excess of joy does not imply that there's something "wrong" with (for instance) having a good, long, hearty laugh with friends; but if you find yourself joking and laughing all the time—even when nothing is funny to others in the room—you may have an imbalance of the fire element. The heart and small intestines are organs connected to the fire element. According to TCM, it means that these organs are handling more of the effects of the Fire imbalances of the body than the other organs.

Also according to ancient Chinese medicine, your liver (which governs or carries your anger) gets out of balance when you are angry; anxiety, guilt and fear take energy away from the kidneys, and excessive sadness and grief can be an indication of an imbalance of the lungs or large intestine. The key is to avoid unnecessary extremes.

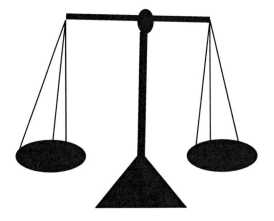

Maat/Equilibrium

Meditation

When you are in your personal space of equilibrium, you feel the need for nothing. You have ameliorated and therefore quieted your addictions, thus rendering them ineffective in their attempts to sway you out of balance; everything is in its comfort zone; your energy is no longer spent in useless attempts to justify the actions once generated by those now-defunct addictions, and you are in a state of healing and preservation.

Total equilibrium is not something we achieve or "get", for that would be perfection, and with perfection not only are we no longer compelled by the forces of duality that create the imbalances in this consciousness paradigm, but we would have no reason for remaining in this present physical state. (This doesn't nullify our previous statements regarding perfection; yes you are still perfect, with your imperfections☺

Meditation along with the practice of all 7 Steps to Wellness and Healing can help bring you to your own personal still-point of equilibrium. Like fasting, it is also a valuable instrument that actually incorporates several of the 7 Steps to Healing at one time. With meditation we release thoughts of the past and future while focusing on the immediate present; we raise our spiritual and physiological vibrations to a level where all aspects of our 'Triune Self' resonate in agreement together, as we are able to bring ourselves into a more balanced, peaceful state of mind.

There are different forms of meditation—some more "formal" than others, but they all help to improve our state of being.

"Meditation brings wisdom; lack of meditation leaves ignorance. Know well what leads you forward and what holds you back, and choose the path that leads to wisdom."

- Buddha

In today's society we think we don't have time to meditate, partially because we don't know how to realistically incorporate it into our already too busy schedules. Nevertheless, when we take just a few minutes a day to be still and turn our attention inward, we can realize even more than a peaceful state of being (as if that weren't enough!). We can focus on the inner light within, re-connect with the Breath of Life, release anxiety and other negative energies and establish new personal agreements, all through daily focused meditation.

It is a well-known fact (in certain circles) that meditation will cause one to increase alpha-wave brain activity (associated with deep relaxation), and in those who have practiced for several years, a considerable increase in theta-wave activity (associated with a deep, healing sleep-state) while simultaneously involving many neurons firing synchronously. But more recently, studies at Yale, Harvard, MIT and the University of Wisconsin have found that regular meditation can actually alter the physical structure of our brain matter, slightly increasing the thickness of the cortex, allowing for improved cognitive function. In other words, meditation is a special type of exercise of and for the brain that will "build it up" (in a manner of speaking) and increase your capacity for learning.

Again, to assist in your quest for equilibrium, find a little time for meditation – even if you have to get up a little earlier in the morning; go to bed earlier in the evening or take a few minutes of a lunch break. Whatever it takes for you; you will find your own way, and you'll be so glad you did.

"*The coordinated physiological processes which maintain most of the steady states in the organism are so complex and so peculiar to living beings - involving, as they may, the brain and nerves, the heart, lungs, kidneys and spleen, all working cooperatively-- that I have suggested a special designation for these states, Homeostasis. The word does not imply something set and immobile, stagnation. It means a condition-- a condition which may vary, but which is relatively constant.*

It seems not impossible that the means employed by the more highly evolved animals for preserving uniform and stable their internal economy (i.e., for preserving homeostasis) may present some general principles for the establishment, regulation and control of steady states, that would be suggestive for other kinds of organization even social and industrial- - which suffer from distressing perturbations.

Perhaps a comparative study would show that every complex organization must have more or less effective self-righting adjustments in order to prevent a check on its functions or a rapid disintegration of its parts when it is subjected to stress. And it may be that an examination of the self-righting methods employed in the more complex living beings may offer hints for improving and perfecting the methods which still operate inefficiently and unsatisfactorily."

Walter B. Cannon, Wisdom of the Body, 1932

Since 1932, **Homeostasis** has been one of the many terms we use to represent physical, internal equilibrium and define wellness. It is the steady state of balance that your body is constantly seeking as it performs literally hundreds of actions to achieve it. Below are just a few of the ways it demonstrates homeostatic action...

Sodium/Potassium Gate - Every cell in your body has a way of generating energy, based on a 2 to 1 ratio of sodium to potassium. To maintain homeostasis, more sodium is needed outside the cell, while more potassium is necessary within. When there is either too much or not enough of one of those (electrolyte) minerals in your extra-cellular fluid (ECF), the cell wall actually opens its "gate", and allows a transfer that brings the ratio back to 2 to 1.

Thermoregulation - Our bodies seek to maintain a temperature of 98.6 degrees Fahrenheit. When it exceeds this temperature your heart and lungs increase activity and you perspire to cool off. Inner Intelligence also detects rampant, infectious bacteria, and raises the body temperature (fever) to eliminate it.

PH – (Potential Hydrogen) Different areas of the body require varying levels of acid or alkalinity to maintain a proper chemical balance.

For the equilibrium of life to be chemically maintained, the blood pH must be in a narrow range of 7.3 to 7.45; if it rises above 7.8 (too alkaline) or drops below 6.8 (too acid), death can occur.

The kidneys main function is to filter out harmful acidic particles. To assist the kidneys, we create and dissolve various chemical solutions of electrolyte minerals called "buffers" into the bloodstream that also help regulate blood pH.

The lungs bring oxygen, which is alkaline, and expel carbon dioxide, which is acidic.

The endocrine glands – pituitary, adrenal and others – secrete hormones that affect and regulate every function in the body.

The exocrine glands – digestive, salivary, sweat – create secretions that leave the body.

Brain/cellular interface- The brain determines when and where there is a discrepancy that threatens homeostasis—for itself, (neuronal homeostasis) as well as in the body, in many different ways. Drinking sufficient amounts of water is one way to ensure that we have the hydro-electric energy in the cells to carry out the various tasks required for this process.

.

Our electromagnetic field levels determine the conditions for homeostasis for the above listed chemical activities. As I said before, the body incorporates hundreds of processes to achieve homeostasis, thus assuring the biological equilibrium necessary for healthy life.

Of course, none of these actions are without a spiritual component.

In the beginning of chapter one I said that when you are well your personal consciousness rests in a space of equilibrium. Now that we've briefly discussed the many aspects of equilibrium, remember also that the exercise of one's awareness occurs on many levels. Take for instance, the precursory activities of thought, and its journey through the labyrinths of the mind into a physical expression.

Before the initial spark of an innermost conceptual inkling is recognized and eventually unfolded by thought, (like a nagging question that begs to be answered) an unexpressed aspect of the Will creates an infinitesimal microcosmic vacuum. Within that very moment, the Will is being qualified by overt conscious thoughts, judgments, emotions and feelings; the true self, that is, the "real" you, is already aware of what you may not yet consciously recognize, and issues a "request" on your behalf; this request, whether the response is to your benefit or to your detriment, is one that the Universe is compelled to satisfy. Now enter the photonic particles from within waves of light, propelled by intent, reconciling all the varying frequencies of your mind, cells and spirit, until they all balance in agreement with the request issued.

The result is the physical manifestation of a metaphysical process of the mind—an expression of Maat, equilibrium or dis-ease, between the visible and invisible worlds of being. Again, the metaphysical (or spiritual) is the template for every plane of physical existence.

When atoms, molecules, tissues, organs, muscles and bones respond in agreement with the above-mentioned events that encourage wellness, you are expressing the Universal principle of Maat/equilibrium, and when the spirit/emotions, atoms, et al disagree, the body will invariably reflect the inevitable consequences of dis-equilibrium.

"The best doctors in the world are Doctor Diet, Doctor Quiet, and Doctor Merryman."

- Jonathan Swift (1667-1745)

Nutrition and Equilibrium

Since we have already discussed several aspects of good nutrition, and since our focus on the 7 Steps to Healing and Wellness is broader than one of diet alone, this section will be brief.

It is (of course) important to have sufficient nutritional support to assist in the process of sustaining mental, emotional, as well as biological equilibrium. Besides the biological concerns, we often don't realize the kind of impact nutrition can have on our mental, emotional and spiritual existence. This is especially important for the developing minds of children. (My book entitled *Dietary Child Abuse— Are you Unknowingly Guilty?* on children and nutrition will extensively explore this matter)

One example that can demonstrate the impact of nutrition on our mental ability is the use of essential fatty acids (EFA's). All fats have fatty acids, but not all fats are considered essential. Essential fatty acids are polyunsaturated, cannot be created by the body, and therefore must be included in the diet. Saturated and mono-unsaturated fats are mostly derived from animals, although palm oil is also highly saturated.

Saturated fats become solid when cold or at room temperature, polyunsaturated do not. (I keep my flaxseed and hemp oils in the freezer, and they never become solid.)

There are 3 main types of polyunsaturated fatty acids: the Omega 3 family - Alpha Linolenic Acids, the Omega 6 family - Linoleic Acids, and Omega 9. We tend to get plenty of omega 9, too much omega 6, and not enough omega 3 fatty acids from our diet. These omegas are found in fruits, nuts, seeds, vegetables and fish. Many people believe they must have fish oil to get enough omega-3's, but flaxseed oil has twice as much as is found in fish.

The human brain is comprised of roughly 65 percent fat (and much of that is water). The membrane that surrounds all human cells including those in the brain is a lipid (fat) membrane. The quality of your lipid membranes is largely determined by the quality of the fat that you ingest. Many people who are chronically stressed, depressed, have violent tendencies and show other symptoms of mental disequilibrium suffer from a deficiency of specific omega-3 fatty acids, as well as chronic brain cell dehydration.

When we are under stress, we tend to over produce biochemicals that add even more to the internal stress factor. Linolenic acid—one of the omegas—can slow down the overproduction of stress-inducing biochemicals. Because flaxseed oil is so rich in omega-3 fatty acids, and because it has anti-inflammatory properties, it is now being used with other nutritional factors to replace such harmful drugs as Ritalin. (Ritalin has been widely used for "hyper-active" children since the 1960's)

Incorporating flaxseed oil along with the other components of proper nutrition, sufficient water, proper rest and avoiding emotional extremes, will help you come into the actualization of the fifth Step of personal Equilibrium.

"The most important human endeavor is the striving for morality in our actions. Our inner balance and even our very existence depend on it. Only morality in our actions can give dignity and beauty to life."

\- Albert Einstein

Essential Oil Recommendations

Frankincense (Boswella Carteri)

Often used to help restore emotional balance

Valor

Valor®, the empowering combination of therapeutic-grade essential oils mentioned earlier, works with both the physical and spiritual aspects of the body to increase feelings of strength, courage, and self-esteem in the face of adversity. Renowned for its protective qualities, Valor® enhances an individual's internal resources. It has also been found to help the body self-correct its electrical balance and alignment.

"No diet will remove all the fat from your body because the brain is entirely fat. Without a brain you might look good, but all you could do is run for public office."

- George Bernard Shaw
1856 - 1950

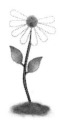

Chapter 7
The Fifth Step

Flow of Life
The Principle of Rhythm

"Everything flows, out and in; everything has its tides; all things rise and fall; the pendulum-swing manifests in everything; the measure of the swing to the right is the measure of the swing to the left; rhythm compensates"

The Kybalion, p35

AFTER SERIOUS CONTEMPLATION OF THE FIRST 4 steps to Healing and Wellness and how they relate to the first 4 principles of the Kybalion, we can easily see how their meanings overlap each other as they all represent slightly different aspects of the One Universal Cosmic Law.

The Principle of Rhythm offers no exception. With it we realize the necessary balancing dynamics between vibrational polarities that create a smooth flow of life. We also understand that just as everything vibrates, everything is in motion.

No situation is stagnant, therefore every situation can and will change. Sometimes the change is quick and obvious, and at other times the change is so slow and gradual that it goes unnoticed for years. If we are observant, we can be more aware of the directional flow of a given circumstance within our lives, and make necessary adjustments to avert an undesired outcome. We can also observe ourselves as though looking from the outside in, and pre-determine the nature and quality of our own personal flow through life.

"Happiness is not a matter of intensity but of balance, order, rhythm and harmony"

- Thomas Merton 1915-1968

While in meditative contemplation, give yourself time to reflect (without judgment) on your own life path. If you have been incorporating the 7 Steps to Healing and Wellness with their corresponding exercises, you will find it easier to observe yourself in your day-to-day inter-action with the world around you.

One of the most difficult aspects of this practice is the ability to observe without judging, so don't be discouraged if you find yourself giving a value to the thoughts that arise. Confirm whether or not you are consistently moving forward toward your predetermined goals, or whether you are tripping and stumbling along your path, only to find yourself "under the circumstances" again and again: "How did I arrive here, and what can I do to avoid a repeat performance? What can I do move forward?"

Here are a few factors that can directly influence your Rhythm, your movement, your "Flow of Life"...

Stress

Stress has become a major contributor to the death tolls of western civilization. It is now the no.1 cause of disease related conditions.

Premature aging, heart attacks, strokes, asthma, high blood pressure, excess weight and insomnia can all be directly linked to and affected by stress. There are different levels of stress; emotional stress is a state that you reach when your brain feels you are threatened or sense danger; the danger you sense can be real or it can be imagined, it makes no difference.

Stress is your internal alarm system at work, reacting to anything that disturbs your equilibrium, and thus your flow; It can cause food to become toxic in the body, acidifying the blood and allowing only a poor absorption of nutrients; stress can cause heart, kidney, and liver dysfunction, loss of the ability to concentrate, high blood pressure, stroke, heart attack, a weakened defense system, and the creation and retention of free radicals. (Free radicals are harmful atomic chemicals with unpaired electrons that need to be paired. They travel through the body, seeking to pair up with others by "stealing" an electron from them, and damaging DNA) One way to look at free radical damage is to think of the rust that occurs when iron and oxygen come together; we call it "oxidative stress".

"I'm an old man and I've had many troubles, most of which never happened"

- Mark Twain

TOLERATION

...the greatest gift of the mind; it requires that same effort of the brain that it takes to balance oneself on a bicycle.

- Helen Keller

Stress is your internal alarm system at work,

Your DNA is a distinct, specific type of amino acid-protein. It consists of oxygen molecules, purine bases, pyrimidine bases, deoxyribose sugar, nucleotides, and nucleosides.

When considering the metaphysical principles of DNA we see that it is a *blueprint of intent* to exist and evolve in this present biological form. That intent is expressed through the dynamics of thought, which effect the day-to-day development and overall bio-spiritual evolution of the DNA. Emotions and intent color and charge the amino acid proteins positioned along the DNA strands, determining (among other things) the rate of vibration the mind and body will express as it participates in the overall flow of life.

Stress and adversity can alter your DNA

"The time to relax is when you don't have time for it"

- Sydney J. Harris

It was once believed that genetics could not be altered after birth. We now know better. There are numerous factors that can have a direct effect on your DNA, and unproductive stress is one of them. (Some types of stress are productive i.e. exercise) Negative stress can also be an initiator of depression.

You have several different ways of dealing with a stressful situation. The most immediate response is usually one that has become automatic; that would be more of a reaction implemented without the benefit of much thought. Your automatic response may appear to be exactly the same as someone else's, but internally—where it really counts—it will be your own unique response, created by your own unique experiences, perceptions and beliefs.

What's even more crucial is the type of atomic vibrations that you create, upon which your photonic waveforms move to foster a series of psycho-spiritual templates. Those templates determine the quality of the blood-matrix from which your cells are nourished.

The sequences of events that constitute your reaction to negative stress can raise the level of acidity in your blood. (Notice I said *your reaction* to stress, not stress alone) Free radicals thrive and proliferate in an acidic environment. And as mentioned before, free radicals can cause DNA damage, as well as a mutation of your cells.

Personal, emotional stress is evidence of the negative (or repressed) emotions we discussed earlier that we use to create a continuous mental loop of perceived threat, anxiety, pain, and consequently our own unique reaction to these three forms of thought.

Man's troubles are rooted in extreme attention to senses, thoughts, and imagination. Attention should be focused internally to experience a quiet body and a calm mind.

- Buddha

"Anger blows out the lamp
of the mind

- Robert Green Ingersoll
1833-1899

Flow of Vital fluids

When you express health and wellness, your vital fluids (blood, craniosacral fluid and lymph) flow without obstructions; your blood cells are not clumping or sticking to the vessel walls; they are freely moving in your blood plasma; the craniosacral fluid encounters no fascial[32] restriction, and the lymph that carries waste away from your cells is not stagnant.

For more than 5 thousand years, Elders of the East have taught the importance of the smooth flow of qi. When you are stressed your qi can stagnate anywhere in your physical body, and will be reflected in your thought processes and your astral body. In many instances, qi gets "stuck" in one or more places, throwing you out of equilibrium, disturbing your flow.

Constipation is another indication of an impediment to your Flow of Life. Not only does it impede your personal physical flow, but it can also be an indication of a deeper impediment to your spiritual flow. When you impede the flow of life emotionally, you will impede the flow of life physically, leading to a tendency towards

---

[32]Fascia = The sheet of connective tissue that surrounds and connect all internal "parts" of the body

constipation. I'm speaking of a chronic pattern here, not of an occasional occurrence.

In your meditations, review in your mind anything, person, emotion or experience that you may be holding on to and refusing to let go.

To help keep your physical elimination processes flowing well, it is more advisable to have plenty of fiber rich fruits and vegetables, and water between meals, than to irritate your colon with laxatives of *any* kind. It's also a good idea for a healthy person to have a colonic once-in-a-while; if you have health issues you will probably need more, according to the advice of your health practitioner. Otherwise, a colonic every 3 months is sufficient—although colonic practitioners will say once a week is better. An enema with plain warm water works wonders!

Be

patient

with yourself

Physical Exercise

Having a sensible exercise program is an excellent way to encourage regularity, and ensure an adequate flow of blood and lymph. Lymph is a body fluid, consisting of water, proteins, cells, waste and fat. It carries foreign protein, lymphocytes (white blood cells), cancer cells, cellular debris and bacteria away from your cells and blood. There are 600-700 lymph nodes in your body; the majority of them are in the abdomen, with another large amount in the neck region. Other major lymph stations are behind the knee, and in the axilla (underarm) and inguinal (groin) areas. Most of us filter about 1 gallon of lymph throughout our bodies every day.

Lymph nodes are small rounded structures, generally located in adipose (fatty) tissue. They have three functions. They are:

1. Filtering stations for noxious matter
2. Production of lymphocytes to fight infections
3. Regulate the concentration of protein in the lymph

My reason for explaining a little about the "lymphatic system" here is to emphasize the importance of regular, daily exercise. You see, lymph has no "pump" like the heart to move it through your body. Though lymph vessels (that network beside your veins to carry the lymph) have their own intrinsic contractility, it is mainly pumped along by the contractions of your skeletal muscles.

In agrarian societies where everyone is working outdoors, using their bodies in manual labor, people don't need to set aside time to exercise; we do. We cannot sit in front of our computers, TV's, and wherever else we sit, and expect our vital body fluids to flow properly; we need consistent, moderate, sensible exercise.

Regular exercise can

- insure proper lymphatic flow
- reduce our chances of premature death
- improve cardiovascular activity
- reduce the risk of diabetes
- reduce the risk of Osteoporosis
- improve digestion and regularity
- raise the pain threshold
- encourage a positive outlook, and
- improve muscular strength.

If you haven't exercised in a long time (3 months or more) or if you have any health concerns at all, consult your health care practitioner before you implement your exercise program. A daily 20-30 minute brisk walk can be a good form of regular exercise.

Dance

Dancing is a form of exercise that can also release stagnant emotional energy, and lift your spirit. The unique joy of personal expression in dance can be a very powerful experience.

It's difficult to be angry or stressed out when you are dancing or singing a pleasant song. Again, it's a matter of choice. Choices become habitual, and habits produce patterns of behavior that create the matrix that sustains your personal flow through life. If you choose to be flexible and less ridged as you come across a rocky road, like water flows, so too will you learn to flow over, under, around and through all obstacles in your path...

Give yourself time to make whatever changes you decide are important or necessary for you. It takes time, patience and consistency to eliminate old habits and create new ones. You may want to join others in an exercise program. I highly recommend belly dancing for women and martial arts for men and women.

The Art of cultural dance ("belly dancing") has become very popular of late. Millennia ago, ancient women of diverse cultures knew it was their duty to teach their young girls the art of being a woman—the conscious ownership of their femininity. Dance was incorporated as a major activity toward that goal; it wasn't labeled "belly dancing", it was just one aspect of the natural order of things. Native cultures used dance not only for entertainment, but also as a means of teaching and solidifying important diverse (historical, familial, etc.) lessons.

Today, it is believed that the form of dance now known as "belly dance" originated in the "Middle East" (as though it is separate from the African continent); let me reiterate that *all* native cultures had a form of feminine dance. It's just that enough resource money and notoriety has been poured into the promotion of the "Middle Eastern" iconic dancer, so as to make her appear to be more authentic—not so.

With all that aside, women across the U.S. are enjoying the benefits of participating in "belly dance classes." One of the greatest benefits is the acceptance of one's own body. I teach belly dance to all sizes and ages of women. They come into my classes with their learned misconceptions and insecurities regarding beauty and their bodies, and before long, they have shed those false self images, and embraced themselves and their classmates; they are no longer ashamed of the size of their bellies, hips—whatever, and they don't feel the need to compare themselves with each other. What a joyful environment in which to get much needed aerobic and strengthening exercise!

To quote Nahida Shiraz, one of my students who has become an exceptional cultural dance teacher in her own right:

"The Beauty Myth: I don't have to tell you, cuz you already know. Just in case you forgot or if you're still thinking you're never going to be skinny enough or blonde enough--well, you know where I'm going with this one. We live in an image-based culture that defines beauty by extremely narrow terms and distorted realities. Shatter the stick-figure image of womanhood and own your beautiful curves cuz this is a Raqs Revolution." [33]

Raqs Sharqi is the Arabic term for "Oriental (Eastern) dance" that many westerners have now become familiar with.

You may or may not want to be a part of the "Raqs Revolution"; you may be shy, and not ready to share the expressive side of your nature.

---

[33] Nahida can be seen on the internet at
http://people.tribe.net/shirazdance/blog/

That's okay, stay at home, but do consider dancing as a part of your wellness program.

Essential Oil Recommendations

(These are some of the EO's that I share with my cultural dance students)

Joy
-a proprietary blend of Rose, Bergamot, Mandarin, Ylang Ylang, Lemon, Geranium, Jasmine, Palmarosa, Roman Chamomile, and Rosewood

Joy produces a magnetic energy to bring joy to the heart. It inspires romance and helps overcome grief and depression.

Release
-a proprietary blend of Ylang Ylang, Lavandin, Geranium, Sandalwood and Blue Tansy

- Helps release anger and memory trauma from the liver in order to create emotional wellbeing, creating a feeling of "letting go".

Essential Oil Recommendations

Peace & Calming
-a proprietary blend of Blue Tansy, Patchouli,
Tangerine, Orange and Ylang Ylang

- Promotes relaxation and a deep sense of peace and emotional well-being; dampens tensions and uplifts spirits; reduces depression, anxiety, stress and insomnia.

Peace & Calming
-a proprietary blend of Blue Tansy, Patchouli,
Tangerine, Orange and Ylang Ylang

- Promotes relaxation and a deep sense of peace and emotional well-being; dampens tensions and uplifts spirits; reduces depression, anxiety, stress and insomnia.

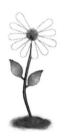

Chapter 8
The Sixth Step
Karma
The Principle of Cause and Effect

"Every cause has its Effect; every Effect has its Cause; everything happens according to law. Chance is but a name for law not recognized; there are planes of causation, but nothing escapes the law."

The Kybalion, p35

KARMA CAN BE DEFINED AS THE SUM EFFECT OF ALL a person has done in the past with what one is presently doing. It is one of the most misunderstood principles of the Universal Law of Cause and Effect. Karma can be looked at in different ways, but the popular view is one that can make you feel a bit helpless. This view says that your karma as fate or luck was established and solidified in a past life, and there's not much you can do to change it. How depressing can *that* be? It's a convenient excuse to stay on the same merry-go-round of unproductive choices and inevitable results—the reasoning being "After all, it's bad karma".

I agree with the approach to Karma is that it is a reality that *can* be changed, and it can also be purposefully and deliberately created. No matter what your Karma has been in the past—even up to this very moment as you read these words— you can change your karma; you need only to fully agree to do so. This is true for everyone. It is the simple realization of Cause and Effect.

The ancient Kemetic elders knew that the energy we send out from our innermost being returns to us within a matching frequency of vibrations. Millennia after this wisdom was passed down from generation to generation, and etched on the pyramid walls; the same principle was repeated in the Holy Teachings of different cultures.

The Christian Bible says "Whatsoever a man sows so shall he reap"[34] ; The Islamic Koran says "Have you considered what you sow?[35]" Buddha says "The kind of seed sown will produce that kind of

---

[34]Galatians 6:7
[35]The Event 56:63

fruit. Those who do good will reap good results. Those who do evil will reap evil results. If you carefully plant a good seed, you will joyfully gather good fruit."

We have seen in the first 5 principles that nothing is in a vacuum. Everything is related to something else; according to Universal Law, things don't "just happen" without a cause.

"For every event that occurs there will follow another event whose existence was caused by the first, and this second event will be pleasant or unpleasant according as its cause was skillful or unskillful." - Buddha

Skillful in this regard, means having been caused by a mental state that is not attached to cravings, clinging, resistance, aversion or delusions. Yogis and students of Yoga offer selfless service to others as a way of paying off past karmic signatures, and creating positive karma for the future. By practicing "Karma Yoga", they exercise the Hermetic principle of Cause and Effect.

The Sanskrit word "Karma" means "to do" or "action". The full expression is "Karma loka" which stands for the plane of action that is desire. As mentioned before in our discussion of Maat/balance/equilibrium, we see again that every thought has its cosmic completion in the universe. Desire plays a major role in the outcome of our thought signatures; the more connected we are to our inner selves, the more conscious we become of our unspoken desires that emanate from within.

In a society that encourages us all towards self-centeredness, superficiality and constant self-gratification, the practice of selfless service is not as easy as it may sound. To do so effectively, we have to consider the underlying motives of our actions, along with the balancing-factor-response to our innate desires, while realizing, acknowledging and releasing our weighty emotional attachments.

("Is that all?"☺)

Although we are not all aspiring Yogis, we all can benefit from the pro-active participation of plotting our own destinies. Every moment of every day, we are creating karmic templates for the future. Fully innerstanding the reality that we are all responsible for our own Karma gives us the confidence we need to be empowered by our own decisions. We can focus on the here and now, as we create metaphysical as well as physical templates for a promising future. We can forgive ourselves for past mistakes and move on, while respectfully allowing others the right to do the same.

"Karma Yoga is the selfless devotion of all inner as well as the outer activities as a Sacrifice to the Lord of all works, offered to the eternal as Master of all the soul's energies and austerities."

- Bhagavad-Gita

My interest is in the future because I am going to spend the rest of my life there.”

- Charles Kettering

Essential Oil Recommendations

Patchouli (Pogostemon Cablin)

Often used to help clarify thought, release obsessions and jealousies

White Angelica

Assists in the release of pent-up negative feelings and restores memories to the point of origin before trauma or anger was experienced

Release

(A blend containing ylang ylang, lavandin, geranium, sandalwood and blue tansy)

Helps release anger and memory trauma from the liver in order to create emotional well-being.

"What would men be without women? Scarce sir, mighty scarce"

\- Mark Twain

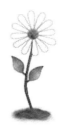

Chapter 9

Step Seven

Posterity

The Principle of Gender

*"Gender is in everything; everything has its
Masculine and Feminine Principles; Gender
manifests on all planes"*

The Kybalion, p39

THE HERMETIC/KEMETIC PRINCIPLE OF GENDER
PROVIDES the basis for a more plenary
overstanding of Polarity, Equilibrium, Cause and
Effect, and indeed, all of the other principles of
the Kybalion. "Gender" is derived from the Latin
root meaning "to beget; to procreate; to generate;
to create; to produce." Studying The Three
Initiate's commentary on Gender will help you to
understand even more thoroughly, the oneness of

the Universe, and the completeness of its synergy. They explain that:

(Gender)"...has a much broader and more general meaning than the term "Sex," the latter referring to the physical distinctions between male and female living things."[36]

They also demonstrate how Gender in its Hermetic sense has been observed by scientists in every entity in all realms of recognizable existence.

Although the duality of sex is merely a manifestation of Gender on only one realm—the organic realm of physicality—it is for our purpose of Health and Wellness, the focus of our discussion.

Many young people today are very confused about Gender and Gender roles, because they receive so much conflicting information. Parents (naturally) teach their children according to their own personal beliefs, which may or may not allow the parents to speak freely on the subject of sex and sexuality; the media seems to have its own agenda related to the Gender issue; politicians argue and legislate to appease one group or the other and "experts" on the subject never seem to

---

[36] The Kybalion, Pg183

have the same opinions, so it remains a blur of mixed messages.

Serious consideration of the effects of societal influence on the principle of Gender deserves much more time and space than we will devote here and now. However, I would like to point out a few relative peculiarities of our society that have a direct bearing on the subject of Gender and its relationship to our Posterity.

A few decades ago, many husbands treated their wives as though they were little children. There was a lot of brutality, abuse and little to no protection or support of any kind for women in those abysmal conditions.
Still, as rampant as this scourge of our society was (and is), it was not as prevalent or widespread as the media would have us believe today.

The gruesome scenarios depicted in the acclaimed book *The Color Purple* by Alice Walker, made popular by the movie that shared its name, and was even made into a Broadway musical (???), was *not* the norm. Let me be clear; *this is in no way an attempt to minimize the painful reality of brutalism experienced behind closed doors against both males and females.* At the same time, I'm reminded of another aspect of historical gender reality seldom spoken of today.

I was born in the 1940's, and grew up in the 50's and 60's. During those years the majority of women were happy to be women. They wanted to marry, to raise a family and be the Queen of their own home. There was also a marked difference between the gender roles in Black families, as opposed those of their White counterparts.

Due to the ever-present, overbearing social disparity in the races, Black families were constantly struggling just to be able to exist on their shamefully reduced incomes, while their White counterparts gratefully cornered the markets of all respected positions, descent salaries and well-paying jobs.

Women in Black families would have *LOVED* to have the homemaker position of their White counterparts. They would have loved to stay home as a "kept woman", with the comfort and security that would have allowed them to be full-time mothers; they would have loved to have spent most of their time at home with their own babies instead of taking care of someone else's, and cleaning someone else's home for shamefully ridiculous pay. But they could not. They were forced by the dynamics of societal of racism to leave their homes and go to work to help support their families.

Then entered the modern feminist movement that "lumped" all women – Black and White together, and pitted men and women against each other in competition. Someone wanted a "battle of the sexes", and seemingly everyone fell for it.

The media has always played a key role in molding *everyone's* worldview, but it is particularly effective in influencing the minds of the young. Today, the media bombards girls and boys with an unrelenting assault on the male gender. In the midst of a powerful, uncontested, unbridled feminist movement, (which we all know was the catalyst for many good and necessary societal changes) television commercials and sitcoms abound not only with insults to the intelligence of the male gender, but even to the fact that men exist. Years ago (particularly in the fifties) the male principle was exonerated and men were presented by movies—and especially TV—as being the head of the family.

In shows like "Father Knows Best", the man was the respected husband and father, and the primary leader in all other aspects of society, while women were portrayed as dutiful wives, loving mothers and homemakers.

Yes, it was an unbalanced approach to dealing with the subject of gender, and yes, there was "I Love Lucy", but at least there was still a modicum of respect for the female principle on TV. - Not so in the reversal of roles today. The male role has been reduced to that of a foolish child.

First there was Homer Simpson, the clueless, degenerate cartoon character on TV, to make us laugh at his incredulous idiocy. Then along came a barrage of other TV characters in dysfunctional families; like the one in the comedic sit-com "Everybody Loves Raymond", where in virtually every episode, Raymond's wife angrily scolds him as she would a child, and he almost apologizes for being alive! These and similar programs bear witness to the now popular practice of passive-aggressive male bashing extant both on and off TV. The serious implications of this anti-male movement are slowly becoming more and more evident, and so will its consequences surely be reflected in the relationships of our future progeny.

Today, you will be "hard pressed" to find a commercial wherein the woman doesn't see all, know all and control all, while the man behaves like a clueless idiot! I've even seen one commercial for a home security alarm system, where a family thought there was an intruder in their home; the father with a fearful look on his face, cowardly cuddled with the children on the bed, while the obviously clear-headed, quick-thinking, fearless mother checked the windows, doors and the alarm system, and called the police.

The pendulum has indeed swung to the farthest extreme. Neither extreme is reflects our Step of Equilibrium. Can we please find the *balance*? What is the message we are sending to our little boys "It's better to grow up to be a woman"?
It would be interesting to get the opinions of young girls and boys on the subject.

Today, special classes for teaching young boys non-violence, and how to respect girls are popping up in major cities as well as small towns. Where are the classes for girls, teaching them to respect boys? Millions of dollars are being commissioned to erect schools and fund special programs for girls only. At the same time millions are allocated for the erection of new prisons to house our boys and young men.

Is this our future?

"Oh, the comfort - the inexpressible comfort of feeling safe with a person - having neither to weigh thoughts nor measure words, but pouring them all right out, just as they are, chaff and grain together; certain that a faithful hand will take and sift them, keep what is worth keeping, and then with the breath of kindness blow the rest away."

- Dinah Craik, 1859

Please try not to allow emotions or preconceived ideas to close your mind to this final Step devoted to our Progeny. It is vital for us all to have a more complete overstanding of the relevancy and consequence of human behavior. Let's be very clear that there is no "right" or "wrong" to be attached to any of the following data regarding homosexuality.

First of all, the principle of Gender is just that – a principle, not a judgment. *No one* has the right to issue judgment—religious dogma notwithstanding. Secondly, not all homosexuality is due to the same causes. It may be convenient, but it is grossly inaccurate to pigeon-hole homosexuals as though they are another breed of humanity, separate from the rest of us (Albeit many homosexuals would like to think of themselves as such.)

"In sex we have the source of man's true connection with the cosmos, and of his servile dependence. The categories of sex are not merely anthropological categories..."

- Nicolai Berdyaev
- 1874-1948

"I am woman! I am invincible!
I am pooped!"

\- Author Unknown

Your children's children are you

This final step to Health & Wellness is not about sexuality. It is in the interest of securing a strong and healthy posterity for several generations through the use of basic, wholistic principles.

Mindful Living, consciously choosing your Agreements, Flowing in peace, Resonating higher vibration frequencies, maintaining Equilibrium and consciously creating your own Karma all culminate to give you the genetic materials with which to create healthy progeny.

Experiencing the Hygienic approach to wellness with adequate nutrition, sunshine, pure water, exercise, loving thoughts and restful sleep from childhood through puberty and the childbearing years will be the foundational insurance that will assist you as you prepare to create a healthy Posterity. Those of us who decide never to have children will still benefit from the information contained this step, because it is based on Divine Universal Principles that positively affect us all.

It is imperative to keep in mind that we are *not* merely the sum of separate body parts. We've become so accustomed to thinking of ourselves as such, that it may be difficult to conceptualize any differing reality.

Despite the use of terms like "digestive system", you really have only one system; the system of light that is you. There is not a single "portion" of you that can function independently from the rest of you. Nevertheless, because we are in a consciousness zone that has limited our purview to the point that it would be very difficult to explain the intricate workings of our existence without the use of such labels, I will use them.

Hormones are chemical messengers that initiate tissue and organ responses. Because they are of a chemical nature, they can easily be affected by other chemicals. Hormones are such powerful substances that extremely minute amounts directly influence *virtually every cell in your body*. Realizing this, you can begin to understand the concerns that natural practitioners have regarding the prodigious amounts of chemicals sprayed on, and packaged into our food today.

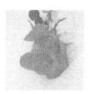

Kids: they dance before they learn
there is anything that isn't music"

\- William Stafford

Hormones work in conjunction with what is called your nervous system, but the effects of hormones on the body can be more prolonged than those of nervous responses. Some hormones will initiate a responsive process that will continue indefinitely. By the way, there are other aspects of your being that also produce hormones. Your stomach, heart, kidneys are among them.

Your ability to reproduce is determined mostly by the aspects of your consciousness called the endocrine and reproductive systems.

Our endocrine system consists of many glands; some of these glands are involved in reproduction, and some are not. From before birth, these glands produce and release into our bloodstream the hormones that dictate the manner in which we will function physically (growth), socially and sexually for the duration of our physical lives.

Estrogen is created predominately in the female body. There are traces of estrogen in the male body as well. It is a powerful amino acid-based hormone that helps the female to develop the menstrual cycle, and grow breasts and the long bones. When too much estrogen is introduced into the bloodstream, it interferes with the integrity of the gender specificity of the male before birth, as a young child, or as an adult. As a result, he will develop breasts; he may also develop a small penis, a low sperm count and a low level of testosterone in his blood.

"Through many sex change procedures we have come to know that a very small dose of estrogen given daily to a fully grown male will result in a fully developed set of breasts, female hips, and loss of facial and body hair. So, even fully-grown males can be fully feminized, at least in outward appearance. This effect would be much stronger on the much smaller body mass of small and growing boys"[37]

The homosexual behavior of Bonobo Apes has become a very popular item as an example of natural Gender ambiguity. Their non-violent demeanor has been attributed to their homosexuality. That's fine—and it may or not be true—but it doesn't change the scientific facts regarding the environment, sex and sexuality.

Testosterone is the chemical polarity of estrogen that helps the male gender distinguish himself from that of the female. It allows him to build larger, denser muscle-mass, grow hair on his face, grow taller, and create sperm. In women, the right balance of testosterone is critical for healthy bones, skin, muscles and sex drive.

---

[37]"Boys Will Be Girls"-truehealth.org

Excessive levels of physical and emotional stress can cause a woman to create an imbalance of testosterone, which can not only cause her to have masculine proclivities, but will also be the precursor to unfavorable health issues—fibroid tumors, hirsutism (unwanted bodily and facial hair), osteoporosis, to name a few.

Endocrine disrupters (ED's mainly in the form of pesticides) are chemical substances that interfere with the natural, normal function of the hypothalamus, pituitary, pineal, thyroid, parathyroid, thymus, adrenal, ovaries and prostate glands (the endocrine "system"). These glands all work together to insure the proper secretions and actions of hormones in the body, which in turn signal any necessary bio-chemical reactions.

ED's sometimes mimic certain hormones, and cause the body to make the right changes at the wrong time (menstruation for 5-year old girls) or the wrong change at the right time (boys growing breasts during puberty). Sometimes ED's replace a healthy signal with one that's too weak to affect a targeted result, such as a diminished growth of the penis; at other times they overwhelm the receptors with a contradictory chemical, causing a cross-gender effect. Endocrine disrupters also cause deficiencies in the body's defenses.

These chemicals not only do damage in the immediate present, but they remain in the blood, affecting DNA, and future generations.

In the 1940's and AGAIN in the 1970's, diethylstilbestrol (DES) an artificial estrogen was prescribed for pregnant women for the prevention of miscarriages. Generations later, DES was found to be the cause of millions of cervical cancer cases of the *daughters* of the original women who were given DES.

Phytoestrogens are naturally occurring compounds in certain plants (vegetables) that can mimic estrogen in the body. The two most well known phytoestrogens are the lignans, found in seeds, (flaxseed) nuts and vegetables, and isoflavones, which are abundant in soy.

Soy and the benefits derived from these phytoestrogens have been made very popular in the last decade, but it is highly over-rated. The largest amount of soy used in the United States is genetically modified; it is not the same chemical compound that the Japanese and Chinese have used for generations; they use a more organic, natural form of soy, and they use much less of it, in comparison to the amounts used in the U.S. The wild soybean *Glycine soja*, found in north-eastern parts of China, the former USSR, Korea, Taiwan and Japan, and which *could contain very little to no isoflavones at all,* is not what we are getting when we buy soy products today. Now we have Glycine Max, which has been cultivated to maximize financial profit[38], and is loaded with soy isoflavones. If you do a research study on soy isoflavones, you'll find a plethora of data touting its wonderful benefits; but when you look deeper, you'll find that that data is dubious at best. The Glycine Max soybean has not been used long enough for us to have sufficient data as to its safety. Statements by soybean manufacturers that claim *"... isoflavones have been consumed by millions of humans for over two thousand years"* have not—and cannot yet be substantiated.

An article by Dr. Mike Fitzpatrick, PhD, MNZIC, was submitted to the FDA in an effort to block inclusion of isoflavones, in the GRAS (Generally Recognized as Safe) list of ingredients in foods and medicines. In it he states:

"Until more extensive epidemiological studies are undertaken with clearly identified endpoints (such as breast cancer, thyroid disease or immune system dysfunction) it must be concluded that

---

[38] According to the American Soybean Association, 85.5 million metric tons of soybeans were harvested in the United States in 2004.

there is no certainty that soy isoflavones are safe at all."[39]

My remaining comments regarding soy are directed at the use of genetically modified (GM) soy, and Glycine Max. Not the original wild soybean.

There are many draw-backs to the use of soy that until recently, have remained concealed from the public (due to powerful lobbying on the part of State Soybean Boards).[40]   Even now, a majority of shoppers believe that ingesting lots of soy is "good for you", when the reverse is true. This can really be a problem for vegetarians; too many vegetarians consume way too much of too many soy products. They eat tofu (soy) burgers, tofu franks, tofu "chicken", soy cereal, soy cookies, soy ice cream, soy chips and other highly processed, artificial foods. They drink lots of soy milk, and soy protein drinks, all the while, thinking they are healthier than meat eaters; but "It ain't necessarily so".

As to how soy can negatively affect our Progeny, I'll just mention a few points:

---

[39] A copy of this article can be seen on the website of the Weston-Price Foundation.
[40] Economics has almost total precedence over efficacy in the health and medical industries.

- Soy can cause developmental disorders, behavioral disorders and cancer.
- Soy-based "milk" formulas have been directly linked to autoimmune thyroid diseases in infants.
- Soy phytoestrogens can cause infertility and breast cancer in men and women.

Pseudo-estrogens are plant based steroid compounds that are often identical to phytoestrogens. Sometimes they differ in that they have a more man-made chemical constitution, but they interact in the mix of chemical metabolism in our bodies in just the same ways.

These chemical compounds that contaminate our food come from several sources.

"Once you change the development of an organ there is no way to undo that effect. It's a life sentence -- that's a lifetime consequence. Medical science can't undo the development of organs."

- Fredrick Von Saal, Professor of Biological Sciences, University of Missouri

Dr. J Robert Hatherill writes:

"Because we have failed to quickly distinguish the side effects of industrial chemicals, we have been bathing in a sea of estrogen-like compounds. Many items with vastly different chemical structures... can mimic the female hormone estrogen... PCB's[41] have recently been linked to depressed immune systems, and even to reduced fertility in males ...In Florida, alligators have penises so short they cannot fertilize female alligators. In California, lesbian gulls on Santa Barbara Island resulted when low levels of DDT were introduced into gull eggs.
Environmental chemicals show the same kinds of results in altering male reproductive processes. PCB's are linked to a 50% reduction in sperm counts during the last century in men from industrialized countries!
A study in Taiwan showed that males exposed to PCB's while in their mother's wombs developed smaller penises when they matured, compared to normal Taiwanese males...[42]

Household pesticides, plastic containers, sunscreen agents, florescent lighting and baby bottles are a few more examples of how pseudo-

---

[41]polychlorinated biphenyls

[42]Eat to Beat Cancer, J Robert Hatherill; pages 43, 45.

estrogens can make their way into our homes and into our bodies. PCB's are generously sprayed on farm vegetables; farm raised salmon also has extremely high levels of PCB's (along with sea lice, food dyes, DDT, and a few other choice poisons). These chemical agents have a more potent effect in infants and children than they do in adults, due to the increase in ratio of chemical-to-blood in their smaller bodies.

In an Abstract entitled *Epigenetics, Evolution, Endocrine Disruption, Health, and Disease,* biologists David Crew and John A. McLachan write:

"Endocrine-disrupting chemicals (EDCs) in the environment have been linked to human health and disease. This is particularly evident in compounds that mimic the effects of estrogens. Exposure to EDCs early in life can increase risk levels of compromised physical and mental health. Epigenetic[43] mechanisms have been implicated in this process.

---

1. [43]Epigenetic – an entity developed by successive differentiation of an unstructured egg rather than by a simple enlarging of a preformed entity.

Another source of estrogen is (believe it or not) our drinking water. It is a known fact that our water is re-cycled. That is, water that is flushed as waste from women who use birth control pills eventually returns "purified" to our faucets. The current water purification process is not efficient enough to eliminate the estrogen compounds.

According to the United States Geological Survey (USGS) taken in 2005, USGS scientists sampled 139 rivers and streams, and found an abundance of xenobiotics (man-made chemicals) from literally hundreds of prescription and over-the-counter drugs and personal care products lingering in our water supply. This is only one route high dosages of pseudo-estrogens and other pollutants take to end up in our water supply.

Unfiltered, unpurified water has become a carrier of chlorinated carcinogenic compounds called "trihalomethanes" (THMs). THMs are released into the air when we are showering[44] or bathing, washing dishes, and flushing the toilet.

When inhaled or ingested, THMs accumulate in the fat cells, and chemically bind with and damage DNA. Additional information regarding chlorine and trihalomethanes research is noted in

---

[44] A shower-head water filter is a good solution here. You can get an excellent one from cmorrison.qhealthzone.com

the *Essential Oils Desk Reference,* where it reports:

"A California Department of Health study surveyed 5,144 pregnant women to determine the effects of THMs in the drinking water (Waller et al., 1998). ...They found that pregnant women who consumed more than 5 glasses of water a day containing more than 75ppb (parts per billion) had double the risk of spontaneous abortion.)"

and again, in a study conducted in North Carolina

"...They found that women who suffered the highest amounts of exposure to THM in the drinking water had almost triple the risk of miscarriage."

The principle of Gender is being directly affected and manipulated by the chemicals we have introduced into the environment.

Sources of harmful endocrine disrupters include non-organic vegetables, fish, red meat, chicken, pork, turkey, eggs, and non-organic dairy products. As a result we are experiencing an over-dose of estrogen being introduced to the general population, and a spiraling decrease in the levels of testosterone in our men.

You may have wondered why the huge and still growing demand for sexual enhancement drugs for both male and female has surfaced in the last decade. Low testosterone coupled with high estrogen in men, and increasing testosterone with low estradiol (an estrogen precursor) in women play a major role.[45] These abnormal percentage levels of hormones also add to the growing infertility problem that many specialist doctors are treating today, on several continents.

So far, we've discussed the effects of only a few endocrine disrupting chemical compounds (DDT, PCB's, pseudo-estrogens) as they can impact our ability to reproduce. What significance can this have regarding Progeny, our 7th Step to Wellness?

---

[45] Again, "The Wounded Womb" will give more insight into this issue.

"The main difference between men and women is that men are lunatics and women are idiots."

\- Rebecca West
1892-1983

It is just as important for males to have healthy bodies with which to produce sperm as it is for females to have healthy bodies to produce healthy eggs and placentas. Obviously, it is the mother who nourishes the unborn progeny from conception until birth (and hopefully with nutritious breast milk, for at least 6 to 18 months). But the literal spark that initiates new life comes from the father. It is the sperm of the father that determines the gender of the coming child. His DNA will transfer his strengths, weaknesses and proclivities down to subsequent generations.

DNA is fragile; when in the process of dividing, the surfaces of DNA molecules are more vulnerable to damage and/or mutation. Infants and children are far more susceptible to DNA damage, because they are growing. Their DNA is always rapidly dividing. As mentioned before, we can purposefully affect our DNA by supplying our bloodstream with pure water, higher vibrational thinking and good nutrition, with which to bathe our DNA strands. Avoiding harmful chemicals will help us to protect the DNA, and re-enforce our practice of healthy living.

Our nutritional requirements on molecular and cellular levels may seem to be complex, but we can take care of those needs by adhering to very basic and simple guidelines.

Again, I emphasize the importance of ingesting organic food as opposed to that which is non-organic. It's not just the crops that receive the harmful chemicals; it's the already depleted soil that is also the recipient of the highly noxious chemical spraying—along with artificial fertilizers—season after season, year after year. The fact of the matter is that the entire ecosystem is grossly affected by this practice. We may never know the full extent of the damage caused by the chemical poisoning of the environment. But we do know that it is a direct cause of endocrine disorders.

The Hermetic Principle of Gender guides us to consider our Posterity for many generations to come. By reflecting on what our thoughts, intentions and actions have given us so far, we can make a conscious agreement to slow down the chemical mat truck that's speeding down the hill towards inevitable catastrophe; or we can choose to ignore the overwhelming evidence of chemical use gone haywire, and continue to wonder why 5 year old girls are menstruating, boys are growing breasts, young couples can't have children and our overall life expectancy isn't really improving.

As we have seen repeatedly throughout our discussion, everything is governed by the law of

Cause and Effect; everything is a matter of choice.

Essential Oil Recommendations

Longevity

A proprietary blend of Clove, Orange, Thyme and Frankincense

-Contains high amounts of DNA protecting oils with high antioxidants action. Prevents premature aging

Mister

A proprietary blend of Yarrow, Sage, Myrtle, Fennel, Lavender and Peppermint

-Helps to decongest the prostate and promote greater male hormonal balance

Essential Oil Recommendations

SclarEssence

A proprietary blend of Clary Sage, Peppermint, Sage Lavender and Fennel

-Balances female hormones naturally with essential oil phytoestrogens

Hope

A proprietary blend of Melissa, Spruce, Juniper and Myrrh

-This blend helps to reconnect with a feeling of strength and grounding, restoring hope for tomorrow

"It does not take much strength to do things, but it requires great strength to decide what to do."

- Elbert Hubbard *(1856-1915)*

Summary

There is nothing you can take that will heal you. Consider Therapeutic Essential Oils and Juice Plus+ as wonderful gifts that will assist in the healing process, but **you are your own healer.**

The Kybalion in its entirety is far more profound than this discussion on Health, Healing and Wellness can express; but its universal principles of transmutation do lend themselves perfectly to our 7 Steps toward holistic personal advancement.

Remember:

1. *"THE ALL is MIND; the Universe is Mental'*
Mindful Living enables us to free ourselves of weighty, emotional baggage, and allows us to be content to live fully in the present.

2. *"As above, so below; as below so above."*
Whatever you **Agree** to with your mind, you will reflect in the actions of your body.

3. *"...Everything is in motion'; everything vibrates'; nothing is at rest."*
You can raise your vibration frequency to **Resonate** on higher planes of consciousness.

4. "Everything is dual'; 'everything has two poles; everything has its pair of opposites."
Through Hygienic principles of Health, we can balance our lives, just as our internal bodies are constantly seeking **Equilibrium**.

5. "Everything flows, out and in; everything has its tides..."
Be conscious of the many tools at your disposal, to assist in your quest for a smooth **Flow of Life**.

6. "Every cause has its Effect; every Effect has its Cause; everything happens according to law."
You *can* plot your own destiny, and create your own **Karma**.

7. "Gender is in everything; everything has its Masculine and Feminine Principles."
Let's make the necessary environmental and societal agreements, changes and choices that will be good for the sake of **Posterity.**

Looking back to the days when our ancestors, the first Hygienicists, actually breathed pure air, drank pure water, ate pure, clean, raw foods, walked, ran and flew (using their minds and bodies only—not airplanes) where they wanted to go, "drank" in the sun, traversed the planets, and were spiritually connected with the universes, we can readily see how they lived to be 700, 800 and 900 years of age.

What we have today is not health as it was then. Every 10 years or so, we lower the standards; we keep lowering the standards, and re-defining the parameters of what constitutes health, to suit our fantasy of latter day progress and superiority over the native peoples of the world—you know who I mean, the ignorant one's who are depicted on the "History" Channel (quotations carry a great deal of sarcasm here—*that's* another subject altogether!) That's fine—if that's what we want to do—if we just "want ours now", and don't necessarily care about what our children's children will experience. But if we, like the so-called Native Americans who plan their lives to benefit 7 generations, DO care about the future, we need to start behaving like we do.

Globally, we have a lot of work ahead of us, (beginning with consciousness rising) to restore our planet to the life sustaining condition it once was, but it's not an impossible endeavor. It's a monumental task, but it can be done. We can start on an individual basis, using the 7 Steps to re-establish vibrant health in ourselves, our families and our communities, and then ultimately connect spiritual and cultural agreements with those of like mind throughout the world.

I sincerely wish for you ankh, udja, snb nfr[46]

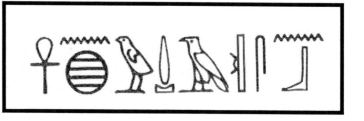

(Life, Prosperity, and Good Health)

---

[46] Ancient Kemetian words of Mdw Ntr

About the author

Nalani Valentine CND, PhD, (known as Dr. Nalani), is a Naturopathic Doctor of the Hygienic Sciences, and a Priestess after the order of the Kemetian Mystery System. She is the founder of the *Heal by Touch Wellness Oasis*, Co-Director of *The Self-Healing Education Center* in New York City, and Co-founder of *The University of Kemetian Sciences Online.* She is also a nationally certified New York State Licensed Massage Therapist, a member of the *American Massage Therapy Association* and the *International Association of Colour Therapy (IAC).*

Dr Nalani holds a Master of Science in Education, a Doctorate in Classical Naturopathy, and a PhD in Hygienic Science.

In 1996, Dr. Nalani was diagnosed with breast cancer. She healed herself, using the same principles that are in her book, *7 Steps to Healing and Wellness, Using the Kybalion as a Guide*, without the use of pharmaceutical medication, and has been cancer-free ever since.

In 1977 she began her 30 year language career as an Interpreter of American Sign Language (ASL). In 5 years, she was teaching ASL for several CUNY colleges in New York City, and subsequently, at the Seymour Joseph Institute of American Sign Language, also in New York where she taught ASL, as well as the advanced level of their Sign Language Interpreting program.

Her studies in Mdw Ntr (pronounced "Medu Netcher) commenced in 1998 with Mfundishi Jhutyms Salim, and continued with Dr. Rkhty Amen Jones, renowned Linguist, Egyptologist and Founder of the Institute of Kemetic Philology.

Between her lecture-tours across the United States and London, UK, and handling administration of the University of Kemetian Sciences, Dr. Nalani partners with her husband Dr. Phil Valentine, in online Wellness Consulting.

Web sites:

www.templehealing.com
www.healbytouch.com
www.uksnow.org
www.lulu.com/content/395457

Contact:
drnalani@healbytouch.com
info@healbytouch.com
info@kemetaphysics.org

By telephone (office): 386.456.9279

CPSIA information can be obtained at www.ICGtesting.com
Printed in the USA
BVOW040056070613

322489BV00004B/587/P